NOVEL ANGIOGENIC MECHANISMS

ADVANCES IN EXPERIMENTAL MEDICINE AND BIOLOGY

Recent Volumes in this Series

NOVEL ANGIOGENIC MECHANISMS

Role of Circulating Progenitor Endothelial Cells

Edited by

Nicanor I. Moldovan, Ph.D.
The Ohio State University
Columbus, Ohio

Kluwer Academic / Plenum Publishers
New York, Boston, Dordrecht, London, Moscow

Library of Congress Cataloging-in-Publication Data

International Workshop "Novel Angiogenic Mechanisms" (2002: Columbus, Ohio)
    Novel angiogenic mechanisms: role of circulating progenitor endothelial cells/edited by
Nicanor I. Moldovan.
      p.   cm. — (Advances in experimental medicine and biology; v. 522)
    Proceedings of an international workshop held on April 16–17, 2002 in Columbus, Ohio.
    Includes bibliographical references and index.
    ISBN 0-306-47697-5
      1. Vascular endothelium—Congresses.   2. Neovascularization—Congresses.   3. Stem
cells—Congresses. I. Moldovan, Nicanor I. II. Title. III. Advances in experimenatl
medicine and biology; v. 522.
      [DNLM: 1. Neovascularization, Phyiologic—Congresses. 2. Angiogeneis
Factor—Congresses. 3. Endothelial Growth Factors—Congresses. WG 500 I615n 2003]
    QP110.V34 I56 2002
    612.1'3—dc21

                                  2002043276

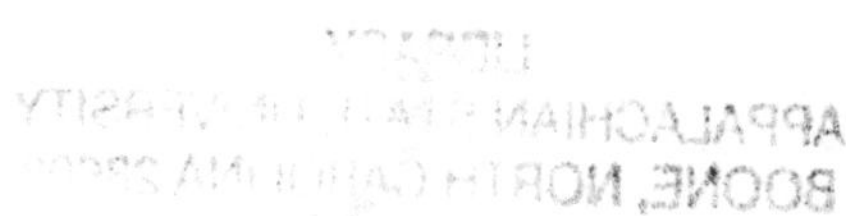

Proceedings of the International Workshop "Novel Angiogenic Mechanisms," held at Davis Heart and Lung Research Institute in Columbus, OH, USA, on April 16–17, 2002.

ISBN 0-306-47697-5

©2003 Kluwer Academic / Plenum Publishers, New York
233 Spring Street, New York, New York 10013

http://www.wkap.nl/

10 9 8 7 6 5 4 3 2 1

A C.I.P. record for this book is available from the Library of Congress

Printed in the United States of America

FOREWORD

New experimental observations often require fresh concepts for their interpretation, and at times even changes of paradigms. This is the situation with the recent realization that circulating endothelial progenitor cells may have an important contribution to the maintenance and formation of new endothelium in adult organisms, in a surprisingly wide variety of situations. The classical paradigm of angiogenesis, centered on the notion of "sprouting" can hardly accommodate them. It was previously realized that it needs to be "stretched out" to include alternative mechanisms of microvascular development, such as intussusception and capillary fusion. However, a major debate where to reconsider the sprouting mechanism, and to promote alternative views, did not take place yet. The number of publications in this field increased exponentially in the last years. Nevertheless, the concepts and notions so much needed to describe and to explain the new observations are still scarce, and heterogeneous.

Within the larger community dedicated to the study of angiogenesis, the researchers involved in investigation of circulating precursor endothelial cells biology represent a subgroup with specific preoccupations and opinions. Many of them did not meet each other so far, and no major scientific events have been dedicated before exclusively to their interests.

For the above reasons, the idea to organize a symposium addressing the new developments in angiogenesis research was received with enthusiasm by all those involved in its preparation. This meeting became the International Workshop "Novel Angiogenic Mechanisms", and was held on April 16-17, 2002, in the newly-opened "Dorothy M. Davis" Heart and Lung Research Institute (DHLRI) of the Ohio State University Medical Center in Columbus, Ohio, USA. This institution incorporates a solid interest in angiogenesis and is committed to the support of most advanced developments in cardiovascular and pulmonary medicine, thus it provided an ideal forum for interaction and discussions.

The International Scientific Organizing Committee of the Workshop, which provided constant advice and support, included Dr. Peter H. Burri (Institute of Anatomy, Berne, Switzerland), Dr. Christian C. Hauderschild (Department of Experimental Pathology, J.H. Holland Laboratory, American Red Cross, Rockville, MD, USA), Dr. Klaus Havemann (Institute for Molecular Biology and Tumor Research, Philips-University, Marburg, Germany), and Dr. Nicholas A. Flavahan (DHLRI, The Ohio State University, Columbus, OH, USA).

A special mentioning deserves Dr. Peter Burri, for his enthusiasm and commitment to this meeting from its conception.

During the preparation of the meeting, I received a substantial support from the leadership of DHLRI (Dr. Jay Zweier and Dr. Mark Wewers), Department of Internal Medicine (Dr. Michael Grever), College of Medicine and Public Health (Dr. Fred Sanfilippo), and from the Center for Continuous Medical Education (Mr. Jon Hollet), for which I am very grateful.

The preparation of the workshop benefited from the assistance provided by Melissa Poulos, and could have not be completed without the benevolent participation and total dedication of Mr. Laura Sladoje (Department of Ophthalmology).

Besides DHLRI, the following organizations and companies contributed with funds to the covering of expenses incurred by the meeting: The Ohio State University Office of Research, Gardere, Bio-Rad, Fisher Scientific, Jouan, and Perkin-Elmer.

During the preparation of the workshop and of the manuscript, I received a very much appreciated help from Sumant Kulkarni, MS and from Leni Moldovan, Ph. D.

This monograph contains contributions from the participants to the workshop. I wish to thank them all for their attendance, for the high quality of work presented, for their vivid participation in the debates, and for their willingness to contribute with their presentation-related materials to this proceedings book.

Nicanor I. Moldovan, Ph. D,
Davis Heart and Lung Research Institute,
Columbus, OH, USA.

CONTENTS

NOVEL ANGIOGENIC
MECHANISMS

CURRENT PRIORITIES IN THE RESEARCH OF CIRCULATING PRE-ENDOTHELIAL CELLS

Nicanor I. Moldovan[*]

The papers presented at the International Workshop "Novel Angiogenic Mechanisms" strongly support a role in adult angiogenesis played by circulating cells of various types, in different settings and circumstances (ischemic limbs, retina, heart, bone marrow). The main themes that currently dominate this research field are, among others, the origin of these cells, their phenotypic modulation in vivo and in vitro, their transformation into endothelial cells (EC) and the mechanisms of their contribution to neovessels formation. The workshop illustrated the domain's general lines of investigation and development, for short and medium term. While it is not our intention to summarize here the contributions of the participants, their opinions are cited below, when considered appropriate.

1. NATURE AND DESIGNATION OF CPEC

The nature of circulating cells able to engraft and contribute to the maintenance, repair, or de novo formation of endothelium is still in the process of elucidation (Otani *et al.*, 2002). The unsettled terminology reflects both our limited knowledge, and a true diversity of mechanisms.

Depending on the adopted point of view, *stem*, *progenitor*, and *precursor* were among the suggested designations of the circulating pre-endothelial cells (CPEC). However, these terms are not synonymous. Stem cells are capable of self-renewal. Therefore, those researchers who consider that the CPEC have a true hemangioblast phenotype, in the embryological sense, consider them as "stem" cells (Grant *et al.*, Chap. 5). Others who see the monocytes or the immature dendritic cells as the potential initiators of an endothelial phenotype, do not find the notion of stem cells applicable to their case (Schmeisser *et al.*, Chap. 7), preferring that of *progenitor* cells, and consider

*Davis Heart and Lung Research Institute, The Ohio State University, Columbus, OH, 43210

Novel Angiogenic Mechanisms: Role of Circulating Progenitor Endothelial Cells.
Edited by Nicanor I. Moldovan, Kluwer Academic/Plenum Publishers, 2003.

the presence of stem cells in circulation less significant (Schatteman and Awad, Chap. 2 Havemann *et al.*, Chap. 6).

Nevertheless, this solution has its own difficulties, due to the fact that a progenitor is a cell from which other cell types derive, and it is not known how well this applies for CPEC. *Precursor* was then suggested to be a more appropriate description. However, the monocytes-related CPEC are not, like the precursors, totally committed to become a specific cell type (i. e. endothelial). *Progenitors* seems therefore to be just a reasonable compromise, in between "stem" and "precursors" cells. Even more difficult it is to find a specific term for CPEC derived from monocytes or dendritic cells by a lateral shift of phenotype, similar to trans-differentiation, a possibility strongly supported by in vitro experiments.

Collectively, it emerged that multiple cell types are potentially involved in blood-supported angiogenesis, and alternative mechanisms may contribute to formation of new vessels in the adult organisms. Nevertheless, it is desirable to standardize this terminology, in order to simplify the communication, and to avoid confusions. This task remains a challenge for the future.

2. CPEC MARKERS

Finding appropriate molecular markers is critical for the definition of a "cell type" (Schwartz, 1999). If each cell has had such a signature, then it would be relatively easy to track its origin and its fate, in the process of endothelialization. The strategy would then be to look for endothelial markers among leukocytes, or for leukocyte markers placed in luminal (endothelial) positions.

While this mosaic of characters is indeed empirically found, the interpretation of the data is difficult, because the assignment of the available markers is not unique. For example, CD34+ is a marker for hematopopoietic cells, but at the same time it is a common label of endothelia in vivo (Norton *et al.*, 1993) and in vitro (Mutin *et al.*, 1997). Even the classical marker for monocytes, CD14 is present on some activated EC (Jersman *et al.*, 2001).

Among the cell-specific markers, a distinct category is represented by the activation markers. However, within the new angiogenic paradigm based on CPEC, an "activated" EC found in situ may be an EC modified under the effect of local factors, or, equally well, a CPEC attached to the vessel wall in that position. An indication on what induces a given activation marker traditionally relied on in vitro studies on purified EC cultures, exposed to specific stimulants. However, these studies have their confidence limit set by the in vitro nature of the models, where the complement of genes induced or repressed maybe different from the in vivo counterpart.

It is now well established that the cells may express multiple markers which overlap between different cell types, and that in fact what defines a cell type is not a single marker, but a *spectrum* of surface or internally-expressed molecules (Grant *et al.*, Chap. 5; Schmeisser *et al.*, Chap. 7). We are confronted with a case of fuzzy logic, in its proper sense, where the objects are not uniquely defined but belong to overlapping classes.

The groups of markers used to define CPEC vary depending on the mechanism considered, and on the analyzed compartment. For example, early CPEC may be found within the bone marrow, more mature CPEC in peripheral circulation and those almost converted into EC, in tissues. Early CPEC, phenotypically similar to the hematopoietic stem cells, are supposed to belong to the same group as the CFU-GM cells. With inclusion of the endothelial "stem" cells, the latter would to be better called CFU-GMDE (granulocyte, monocyte, dendritic and EC) (K. Havemann, personal communication). Then, these cells are expected to be positive for the CFU-GM markers (CD34, CD38, CD54 and HLA-DR).

Finding in the circulation cells expressing endothelial markers (von Willebrand factor, Tie-2, etc.) may suggest either newly-formed CPEC not yet incorporated into the endothelium, or EC just detached from it. Therefore, it is not only necessary to test the circulating candidate CEPC for progenitor markers, but also for other (mostly, even though not unique) endothelial-specific *and* non-endothelial molecules.

3. MONOCYTES HETEROGENEITY

Of particular interest is the relationship between CPEC and monocytes. Whatever their phenotype, CPEC belong to the mononuclear leukocytes class, and (because based on function and surface markers they are neither lymphocytes nor NK cells, etc.), by exclusion CPEC could then formally be considered a subpopulation of monocytes, depending on how these cells are defined.

This is not a trivial question because the monocytes are not a uniform cell population. The commonly used marker CD14 is not present uniformly on all monocytes. For example, there is a group of monocytes which are dimly stained with fluorescent antibodies for CD14 antigen, but bright for CD16 (Fcγ-RIII) (Ziegler-Heibrock *et al.*, 1991). These cells are similar in phenotype to the alveolar macrophages, and are estimated to comprise 15% of the human blood monocytes. In the blood a dendritic cells precursor is also present, which is CD14 dim, Cd33$^+$, CD16$^-$ (Szeberenyi *et al.*, 2000). The work done in Dr. Havemann's laboratory has shown that not only monocytes, but the immature dentritic cells as well have the potential to transdifferentiate into EC in vitro (Havemann *et al.*, Chap. 6).

Nevertheless, what the investigators define as *monocytes* are the CD14$^+$, CD45$^+$, and CD34$^-$ mononuclear cells, which have the ability to behave like CPEC both in vivo (Schatteman and Awad, Chap. 2) and in vitro (Schmeisser *et al.*, Chap. 7).

4. THE RELATIONSHIP BETWEEN MONOCYTES/MACROPHAGES AND EC

It was known for a long time that between these two cellular categories there is a special relationship. For embryological, biochemical and functional reasons, they were assigned to the so-called "reticulo-endothelial system" (Havemann *et al.*, Chap. 6). It is believed that about half of the progenitor cells are CD45$^+$. In vitro, even CD 45$^-$ cells over time and in specific conditions, may become CD45$^+$, too. CD14 is not persistent for long time, being lost upon cultivation (A. Schmeisser, round table).

Obviously more in vivo data about CPEC is needed. In the context of the current discussion, it would also be highly informative to re-evaluate the origin of lymphatic, sinusoidal, or spleen EC, and see which markers are shared with macrophages, as well as how and when these makers are expressed (A. Schmeisser, round table).

In order to clarify the direct contribution of monocytes and/or macrophages to EC formation, several strategies are available. One is to analyze the graft re-endothelialization, and see if they are CD45+ or not. In order to track the origin of these cells, they need to be pre-labeled. So far, the fallout endothelialization was analyzed mostly from the point of view of endothelial markers, but less from that of monocytes/macrophages. Ideally, double staining for (re)endothelialization is necessary. In fact this is the weakness of most published papers, an incomplete characterization of cells. Fortunately, new tools are now available, and it will be possible to have circulating cells transgenically expressing various markers like GFP or beta galactosidase, for instance, and used in transplantation and in grafting experiments.

Another related issue is the possibility that mature macrophages trans-differentiate in vitro and possibly in vivo into EC. While the examples of transdifferentiation in general become more and more abundant, the transformation of macrophages into EC is not yet largely accepted (K. Havemann, round table). Experiments to address this question are under way.

5. IN VITRO DIFFERENTIATION OF CPEC

A valuable instrument for assessing the ability of circulating cells to become endothelial is their cultivation in vitro in appropriate conditions. Ongoing research addresses the fate of some of the surface markers during cultivation, both in terms of occurrence, and of disappearance (Havemann *et al.*, Chap. 6; Schmeisser *et al.*, Chap. 7)

An alternative way of tracking the fate of the stem cell-like CPEC is their clonal expansion in vitro. This approach is being currently pursued, and the preliminary data suggest that in appropriate conditions the CPEC may evolve either towards monocytes, or towards EC, but not towards both (E. Gunsilius, round table). This fact does not contradict that the progression of cells trough their developmental phases, in adult as in embryonic animals, is also environmentally controlled (by extracellular matrix, surrounding cells, shear stress, etc).

In fact, recently a single cell-based stochastic model of stem cell maturation, which makes operational the novel concept of within-tissue plasticity, was suggested. It accounts for the hematopoietic stem cell kinetic and functional heterogeneity, reversibility of cellular properties, self-regeneration after damage, fluctuating activity and competition of stem cell clones, as well as the dependency on microenvironment of stem cell quality. In this model, individual cells may reversibly change their actual set of properties within a range of potential options, depending on the influence of the local growth environment. Stochastic switching between the growth environments introduces fluctuations that eventually generate heterogeneity. In this case, stemness is no longer an explicit cellular property, but the result of a dynamic process of self-organization (Roeder and Loeffler, 2002).

6. CPEC MORPHOLOGY

Derived from the difficulty to track the maturation of CPEC by assigning specific markers, the morphological description may become once more very valuable. Efforts should be made to isolate CPEC, analyze them ultrastructurally as fresh isolates, and after controlled culture conditions. FACS analysis alone is not sufficient in this respect. The electron microscopy could say a lot about the morphology and structure of CPEC.

Based on the current understanding, the stem-cell like CPEC may look as small lymphocytes, and those derived from monocytes would have typical monocyte morphology with a wide cytoplasm and a kidney-shaped nucleus. In culture, these cells acquire a heterogeneous morphology, from adherent oval to spindle cells (mixed macrophage/monocyte phenotype). Less adherent small cells, with cytoplasmic extrusions, may later show an endothelial cell morphology.

The stem cells category may also include cells forming colonies or "islands". Usually the cells in the center of the colonies are described as larger than the original or companion mononuclear cells (Kang *et al.*, 2001).

7. ADULT CIRCULATING EC

A renewed attention has been recently given to the distinct class of circulating adult EC (CAEC). These cells have been known for a long time, but the interest for them fluctuated (Schatteman and Awad, Chap. 2). It is considered that CAEC are detached from pre-existent vessels. A likely possibility is that they are shed as early apoptotic EC, and somehow rescued from death, for example by VEGF produced in tumors. CAEC do not seem to derive from bone marrow, because their phenotype is that of mature EC (Mancuso *et al.*, Chap. 9).

However, a maturation process of CPEC taking place in the circulation may also be considered (Moldovan, Chap. 10). The increased number of CAEC found during menstruation can be interpreted either as shedding of EC from pre-existent or damaged vasculature, or as more CPEC mobilized from bone marrow to replace/repair vessels. A kinetic argument is that if the peak of CAEC is at the beginning of menstruation, then they would derive from destroyed vessels; if later, then it is a repair process (P. Burri, round table). The peak is found at the end, thus, this seems indeed a repair process (A. Mancuso, round table).

In myocardial infarction, it was observed a peak of CAEC after several hours, then their number tended to decrease. Because it was reported that stem cells appear at a later stage, after several days, it is interpreted that the adult CAEC are produced in this instance as a consequence of the injury (A. Schmeisser, round table).

8. INTERCELLULAR COMMUNICATION IN CPEC RECRUITMENT AND ENGRAFTMENT

The problem of engraftment of CPEC into the pre-existent endothelium is important, and deserves special consideration. So far only vague hypotheses have been put forward, and there is no model yet which can fully account for the known features of this process.

"Maintenance angiogenesis" is an attractive concept suggesting a role of CPEC in endothelial turnover, by replacing EC lost by apoptosis (Gunsilius, Chap. 3). EC turnover in itself is a territory which needs to be re-explored with modern tools. Apparently it is very hard, if not impossible to see "blank spots" in vivo, probably because the re-covering is very fast. If they were present, clotting should occur within seconds. The replacement of dead EC cells is done with the maintenance of junctional integrity

(Moldovan *et al.*, 1994). It was suggested that blood monocytes may be involved in the removal of apoptotic cells. This does happen in the lung, and it might hold true for other vascular trees as well (P. Burri, round table). Furthermore, the same phagocytes cleaning the debris of apoptotic EC may adhere and fill the empty spots, acquiring EC markers and properties (anticoagulant, among others) and thus become EC surrogates.

As a model of CPEC recruitment, capillary beds may be considered to act as "retention filters" with the ability to slow down, and to retain some of CPEC during each passage (Moldovan, Chap. 10). Thus, during the passage through capillaries, CPEC may have both time and local conditions to mature. If they do not adhere somewhere, they just keep cycling. This would allow the initiation of their differentiation, and suggest an explanation for the gradual transformation of the progenitors in more mature CAEC, rather than derivation from the pre-existent (micro)vascular EC.

More difficult to understand is how, and why, CPEC would incorporate amongst the EC of a close-ended sprouting capillary, or if they rather make their own microvascular tuft. Alternatively, if CPEC have indeed hemangioblast abilities, are they able to form complete blood islands, including erythrocytes and leukocytes? How would they connect to the pre-existing microcirculation? Can they penetrate deeply enough alone in the tissues, or do they need "assistance" from other cell types, such as monocytes/macrophages? The "tunneling" model of CPEC-based angiogenesis was proposed as a possible explanation (Moldovan, Chap. 10).

Data which became recently available suggests a reverse relationship between monocytes and CPEC: the CD14+ monocytes may function as CPEC only in the presence of CD34+ cells (Scatteman and Awad, Chap. 2). The biochemical and cellular bases of this synergism are currently being uncovered by an active research effort.

9. VASCULAR MIMICRY

A general observation made with the CPEC derived from circulating cells is that even when they express EC markers, they may never become "true" EC. This raises the potentially important observation that maybe CPEC contribute functionally to maintenance and repairing processes in the endothelial lining, including formation of pseudo-capillaries, but would remain distinguishable from the native EC.

There are precedents of this type of behavior, namely that of cytotrophoblasts (Damsky and Fisher, 1998). These are fetal cells that cover the maternal blood conduits (the spiral arteries), by replacing the endogenous endothelium, and which acquire an endothelial phenotype (CD31 and anticoagulant surface, among others).

It is debatable at this moment if the "vascular mimicry" of tumor cells falls in the same category. It was shown in some tumors that cancer cells are able to contribute to the endothelialization of blood vessels in their own tumors by creating "mosaic vessels", when bona fide EC are intermixed with tumoral cells in endothelial positions (Chang *et al.*, 2002).

10. CPEC, CLINICAL IMPLICATIONS, AND CELL THERAPY

The practical consequences of mastering the mechanisms of CPEC recruitment and differentiation are considerable. On one side, it may help better understanding the mechanisms of functioning and renewal of healthy tissues, and how these might be modulated in diseases by administration of drugs such as statins (Llevadot *et al.*, 2001; Urlich *et al.*, 2002) or erythropoietin (Ribatti *et al.*, Chap. 4). This opens a whole new avenue of therapeutic angiogenesis, based on cell therapy. Mobilization of bone marrow derived CPEC using VEGF administration is already available (Asahara *et al.*, 1999). Moreover, CPEC can be isolated, expanded din vitro, and re-injected with demonstrated benefit for the ischemic limbs (Schatteman *et al.*, 2000), hearts (Koecher *et al.*, 2001), or retinas (Otani *et al.*, 2002). These are examples of adult "stem cell" based therapy, which make even more questionable the use of embryonic stem cells, at least in an angiogenic context.

11. ACKNOWLEDGEMENTS

The topics of this introduction were addressed by the speakers to the Workshop in their papers, and also in a round table discussion on April 17th, 2002. Participants to this round table were: Peter Burri, Eberhard Gunsilius, Klaus Havemann, Matthias Clauss, Patrizia Mancuso, Nicanor I. Moldovan, A. Schmeisser, and Gina Schatteman.

12. REFERENCES

Asahara, T., Takahashi, T., Masuda, H., Kalka, C., Chen, D., Iwaguro, H., Inai, Y., Silver, M., Isner, J. M., 1999, VEGF contributes to postnatal neovascularization by mobilizing bone marrow-derived endothelial progenitor cells. EMBO J. **18**(14):3964.

Chang, Y. S., di Tomaso, E., McDonald, D. M., Jones, R., Jain, R. K., Munn, L. L., 2000, Mosaic blood vessels in tumors: frequency of cancer cells in contact with flowing blood. Proc Natl Acad Sci U S A Dec 19;97(26):14608.

Damsky, C. H., Fisher, S. J., 1998, Trophoblast pseudo-vasculogenesis: faking it with endothelial adhesion receptors. Curr Opin Cell Biol Oct. **10**(5):660.

Jersmann, H. P., Hii, C. S., Hodge, G. L., Ferrante, A., 2001, Synthesis and surface expression of CD14 by human endothelial cells. Infect Immun **69**(1):479.

Kang, H. J., Kim, S. C., Kim, Y. J., Kim, C. W., Kim, J. G., Ahn, H. S., Park, S. I., Jung, M. H., Choi, B. C., Kimm, K., 2001, Short-term phytohaemagglutinin-activated mononuclear cells induce endothelial progenitor cells from cord blood CD34+ cells. Br J Haematol. **113**(4):962.

Kocher, A. A., Schuster, M. D., Szabolcs, M. J., Takuma, S., Burkhoff, D., Wang, J., Homma, S., Edwards, N. M., Itescu, S., 2001, Neovascularization of ischemic myocardium by human bone-marrow-derived angioblasts prevents cardiomyocyte apoptosis, reduces remodeling and improves cardiac function. Nat Med. **7**(4):430.

Llevadot, J., Murasawa, S., Kureishi, Y., Uchida, S., Masuda, H., Kawamoto, A., Walsh, K., Isner, J. M., Asahara, T., 2001, HMG-CoA reductase inhibitor mobilizes bone marrow-derived endothelial progenitor cells. J Clin Invest. **108(3)**:399.

Moldovan, N. I., Moldovan, L., Simionescu, N., 1994, Binding of vascular anticoagulant alpha (annexin V) to the hypercholesterolemic rabbit aortic intima. An autoradiographic study. Blood. Coag. Fibrinol. **5**:921.

Mutin, M., Dignat-George, F., Sampol, J., 1997, Immunologic phenotype of cultured endothelial cells: quantitative analysis of cell surface molecules. Tissue Antigens **50(5)**:449.

Norton, J., Sloane, J. P., Delia, D., Greaves, M. F., 1993, Reciprocal expression of CD34 and cell adhesion molecule ELAM-1 on vascular endothelium in acute cutaneous graft-versus-host disease. J Pathol. **170(2)**:173.

Otani, A., Kinder, K., Ewalt, K., Otero, F. J., Schimmel, P., Friedlander, M., 2002, Bone marrow-derived stem cells target retinal astrocytes and can promote or inhibit retinal angiogenesis. Nat Med. **8(9)**:1004.

Roeder, I., Loeffler, M., 2002, A novel dynamic model of hematopoietic stem cell organization based on the concept of within-tissue plasticity. Exp Hematol. **30(8)**:853.

Schatteman, G. C., Hanlon, H. D., Jiao, C., Dodds, S. G., Christy, B. A., 2000, Blood-derived angioblasts accelerate blood-flow restoration in diabetic mice. J Clin Invest. **106(4)**:571.

Schwartz, S. M., 1999, The definition of cell type. Circ Res **84(10)**:1234.

Szeberenyi, J. B., Rothe, G., Pallinger, E., Orso, E., Falus, A., Schmitz, G., 2000, Multi-color analysis of monocyte and dendritic cell precursor heterogeneity in whole blood. Immunobiology, **202(1)**:51.

Urbich, C., Dernbach, E., Zeiher, A. M., Dimmeler, S., 2002, Double-edged role of statins in angiogenesis signaling. Circ Res. **90(6)**:737.

Ziegler-Heitbrock, H. W., 1996, Heterogeneity of human blood monocytes: the CD14+ CD16+ subpopulation. Immunol Today, **17(9)**:424.

IN VIVO AND IN VITRO PROPERTIES OF CD34⁺ AND CD14⁺ ENDOTHELIAL CELL PRECURSORS

Gina C. Schatteman, and Ola Awad *

1. CIRCULATING ENDOTHELIAL CELLS: A HISTORICAL PERSPECTIVE

To begin we will briefly describe the history of how we, in collaboration with Jeffrey Isner's group, contributed to the 'rediscovery' of circulating cells that integrate into the endothelium and function as endothelial cells. A number of years ago Dr. Isner and colleagues were studying the effect of vascular endothelial cell growth factor (VEGF) on re-endothelialization of arteries. To test this, they denuded carotid arteries bilaterally and then delivered VEGF protein locally via a double balloon catheter to one of the carotid arteries. Isner and colleagues found that VEGF markedly increased re-endothelialization of the treated artery.[1] However, they also observed that the local delivery of VEGF to one artery improved re-endothelialization of the untreated contralateral artery. Since only small amounts of VEGF were administered, systemic levels of VEGF could not have been appreciably elevated even if none of the VEGF remained at the site of administration. What then might account for the increased contralateral re-endothelialization?

The fact that embryologically the endothelial cells and hematopoietic stem cells are derived from the same precursor, the hemangioblast, suggested one explanation. Perhaps a subset of cells in adult blood maintain this hemangioblastic potential. These circulating cells might be stimulated as they pass through the region of high VEGF concentration in the vicinity of the balloon to take on a more endothelial cell-like phenotype. Such a phenotypic change might also induce the circulating cells to adhere preferentially to sites of denudation where they would fully differentiate into endothelial cells.

A subsequent search of the literature revealed that there was indeed a body of evidence suggesting that endothelial cell or endothelial cell precursors are present in the circulation. In 1932 Hueper and Russel published "Capillary-Like Formations in Tissue Cultures of Leukocytes".[11] One year later "the development of organized vessels in cultures of blood cells", and in 1950 "in vitro blood vessel" formation from bone marrow of adult chickens were described.[16, 30] In addition, reports of 'fallout' endothelialization, i.e.

---

*University of Iowa, Iowa City, IA, 52242.

Novel Angiogenic Mechanisms: Role of Circulating Progenitor Endothelial Cells.
Edited by Nicanor I. Moldovan, Kluwer Academic/Plenum Publishers, 2003.

endothelialization of grafts by blood-derived cells have been appearing almost as long as synthetic arterial grafts have been in use.[e.g.,14, 24, 26, 28] Elegant studies by Sauvage and colleagues showed that when blood flow is present, implanted synthetic arterial grafts can be re-endothelialized even when endothelial cell in-growth from the anastomoses and the vaso vasorum are apparently prevented.[26, 31] Another study found that when bone marrow cells were infiltrated into synthetic vascular grafts, endothelialization occurred more rapidly than in uninfiltrated controls.[15] All of these studies pointed to the presence of endothelial cell or their precursors in the blood, but their identity remained elusive.

2. IDENTIFICATION AND SIGNIFICANCE OF CIRCULATING ENDOTHELIAL CELL STEM CELLS

The putative circulating re-endothelializing cells could be either fully differentiated endothelial cells or they might be endothelial cell precursors. We favored the latter possibility, because earlier reports describing circulating endothelial cells suggested that the cells were both unhealthy and rare.[7, 19, 27] So, if circulating endothelial cell precursors exist, what might their phenotype be? Again we turned to embryology for clues. Hemangioblasts and hematopoietic stem cells can not be distinguished antigenically in the embryo, so we reasoned that an adult hemangioblast should look like a hematopoietic stem cell.

CD34 is an antigen routinely used to enrich for human hematopoietic stem and primitive progenitor cells. Hence, together our laboratories began a search for endothelial cell progenitors among peripheral blood mononuclear cells (PBMCs) enriched for $CD34^+$ cells. Thanks to the tireless efforts of Takayuki Asahara working in Dr. Isner's laboratory as well as the work of a host of others, we demonstrated that $CD34^+$ enriched cells can differentiate into an endothelial-like cell in vitro and incorporate into the neovasculature and express endothelial cell antigens in vivo. [2]

In the years that have followed this work numerous groups using a wide variety of models have shown that a subset of cells in the blood can differentiate into multiple tissue types including blood and endothelial cells.[6, 9, 13, 17] Among cells that are thought to act as stem cells are the $CD34^+$, c-kit$^+$, and sca-1$^+$ expressing and the SP (side population) subpopulations of circulating cells.[8, 12, 17, 25] Each of these cell types is rare in the blood and there is extensive overlap among the populations, so that it appears that true circulating endothelial cell stem cells are rare.

In a study performed in Daniel Bowen-Pope's laboratory on which we collaborated, mice were irradiated to destroy their bone marrow, and the bone marrow was reconstituted with cells from a genetically tagged donor. After allowing the mice to recover for several months, the mice were implanted with a sponge to induce neovascularization. When the sponges were examined subsequently, an average of 10% of cells in the endothelium were donor-derived, suggesting that circulating cells contribute significantly to vascular repair.[3] More recently, Grant and colleagues also reported large scale differentiation and incorporation into the endothelium of bone marrow-derived cells.[9]

3. MONOCYTES AS ENDOTHELIAL CELL PROGENITORS

The high proportion of bone marrow-derived cells in the neo-endothelium seemed remarkable if the aforementioned stem cells are the only source of precursors of endothelial cells in the blood. Thus, we considered the possibility that there might be other circulating endothelial cell precursors. Once again we turned to what is known about the hematopoietic system for clues to their possible identity. Within the hematopoietic system there are both stem and progenitor cells, and there is an orderly progression from stem cell through partially differentiated progenitors to the fully differentiated blood cell. During this process, the various progeny proliferate so that ultimately a single stem cell produces many progenitors and 'fully' differentiated cells. (Fig. 1) For example, cells in the myeloid lineage proliferate as they progress from CFU-GEMM to CFU-GM to CFU-M to monoblast to monocyte before finally differentiating into macrophages or other cells, and while stem cells and CFU-GEMM are rare cells, monocytes represent about 10% of PBMCs. (Fig. 1) If circulating endothelial cell precursors follow the same pattern, there could be a relatively common circulating progenitor.

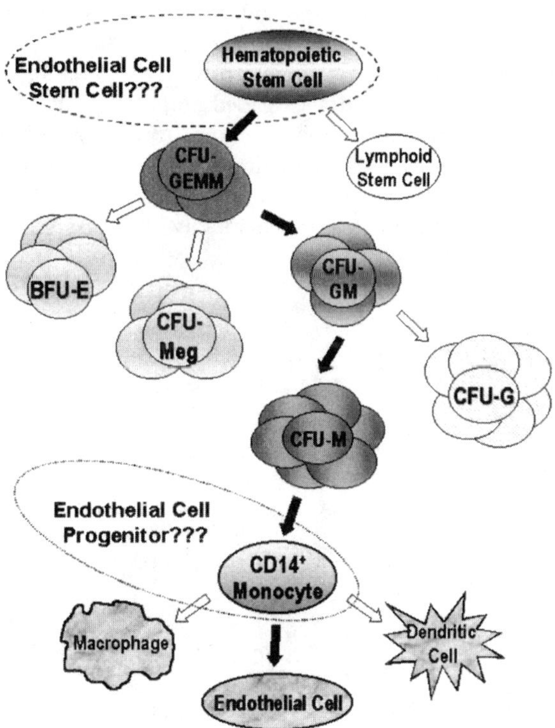

Figure 1. Possible path of endothelial cell stem cell differentiation. Endothelial cell stem cells may be related to hematopoietic stem cells and follow a similar differentiation pathway. They may follow the myeloid lineage path since CD14+ monocytes function as endothelial cell precursors in vitro. Progenitors could be amplified at each stage of differentiation before leaving the bone marrow ultimately releasing large numbers of cells into the bone marrow.

Monocytes seemed to be a likely candidate for endothelial cell progenitor because there appears to be an intimate relationship between monocytes and the endothelial surface during collateral artery growth.[20, 23] Additionally, Waltenberger and colleagues reported that VEGF-A induced chemotaxis is attenuated in monocytes derived from diabetic patients.[29] This is significant because of the association of diabetes with vascular damage and impaired neovascularization. Finally, monocytes are found at all sites of injury and so would be present where and when needed for vascular repair.

To test the hypothesis that monocytes can act as endothelial cell precursors we cultured CD34$^-$CD14$^+$ and CD34$^-$CD14$^-$ PBMCs in conditions that induce differentiation of CD34$^+$ endothelial cell stem cells. Our data indicated that CD34$^-$CD14$^+$ cells differentiated into endothelial cell-like cells, whereas CD34$^-$CD14$^-$ cells failed to differentiate and ultimately died in the same culture conditions. After varying times in culture, the CD34$^-$ CD14$^+$ cells, like their CD34$^+$ counterparts, expressed tie-2, endothelial cell-nitric oxide synthase, VE-cadherin, and low levels of flk-1 and took up acetylated low density lipoproteins. Both Havemann's and Schmeisser's groups have reported similar findings and showed expression of additional endothelial cell antigens on the cells, including von Willebrandt's factor.[4, 22] We and they also reported the ability of the cells to form tube-like structures in vitro.

We observed an additional interesting morphological property of cultured CD34$^-$ CD14$^+$ PBMCs. When cultured at high density for extended periods of time, the cells formed ring-like structures. (Fig. 2) Some lumens appeared to be formed by coalescence of multiple cells. Others were formed by vacuolization similar to what can be observed sporadically in endothelial cell cultures. (Fig. 2A) Over time, small rings tend to fuse creating larger rings. (Fig. 2B-C) These structures look remarkably like cross-sections of

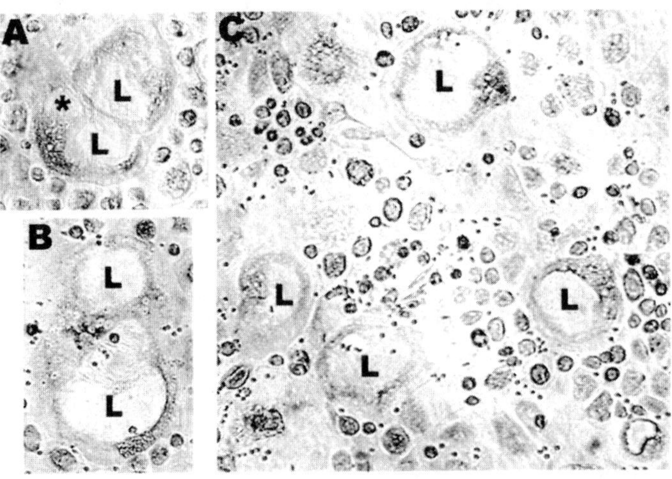

Figure 2. Formation of capillary-like structures by CD34$^-$CD14$^+$ Cells. CD34$^-$CD14$^+$ cells cultured for 24 days on fibronectin in rich medium. A) Three almost fused rings. Ring indicated by * in the lumen is formed by a single endothelial cell. B) Two rings beginning to fuse. C) Area of plate show four discreet rings. L = lumen

capillaries in tissue sections. We have never observed this type of pseudo-capillary formation in any of our endothelial cell cultures. Interestingly, while this phenomena was observed routinely in long-term high density cultures of CD34⁻CD14⁺PBMCs cultures, it was rarely seen in those of CD34⁺ PBMCs.

4. INTER-DEPENDENCE OF CD34⁺ AND CD34⁻CD14⁺ ENDOTHELIAL CELL PRECURSORS

Having established that CD34⁻CD14⁺ cells could take on an endothelial cell-like phenotype in vitro, we next tested the hypothesis that they could also do so in vivo. To this end, an ischemic hindlimb was created in nude mice to induce neovascularization. CD34⁻CD14⁺ enriched cells were labeled with the vital dye, CM-DiI (Molecular Probes, Eugene, OR), and injected intramuscularly into the ischemic limb. In contrast to findings in an earlier study in which injected CM-DiI labeled CD34⁺ cells were observed in the endothelium of the muscle neovasculature, we found no CM-DiI labeled cells in the endothelium five days after injection. However, when unlabeled CD34⁺ and CM-DiI labeled CD34⁻CD14⁺ PBMCs were co-injected into the ischemic limbs of mice, CM-DiI labeled cells were localized in the neovasculature, suggesting that CD34⁺ cells may provide a stimulus for CD34⁻CD14⁺ cell differentiation and/or incorporation into the endothelium.[10] (Fig. 3)

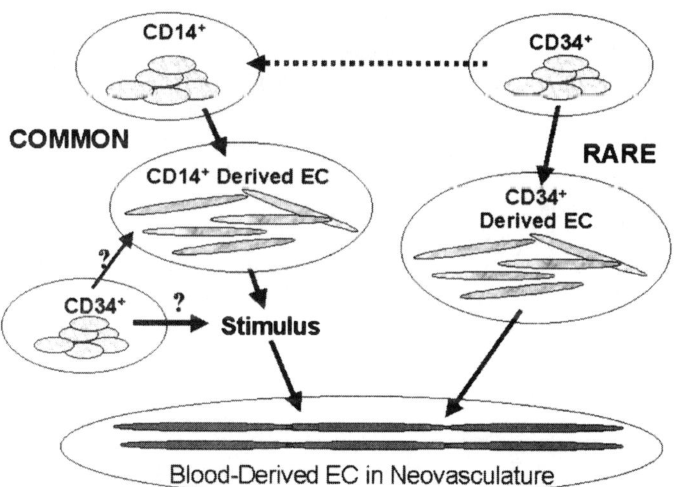

Figure 3. CD14⁺ - CD34⁺ endothelial cell precursor interdependency. CD34⁺ or related cells probably are true stem cells, rarely, if ever, differentiating directly into endothelial cells. Instead, they may produce proliferative progeny which differentiate into CD14⁺ endothelial cell progenitors. Given the appropriate stimulus, CD14⁺ differentiate directly into endothelial cells and incorporate into the endothelium. CD14⁺ cells are probably the most common source of blood-derived endothelial cells. CD34⁺ cells may have a second role as stimulators of progenitor cell differentiation or integration into the vasculature.

What this stimulus is remains to be determined, but there is some evidence that whatever it is may be lacking in diabetic mice. Several years ago we found that while human $CD34^+$ cells not promote revascularization in the ischemic limbs of non-diabetic mice, they profoundly accelerated the restoration of blood flow to the ischemic limbs of diabetic mice. Thus, these non-diabetic derived cells may have provided a stimulus that is present in the non-diabetic but lacking in the diabetic mouse. Of course, there may also be diabetes associated intrinsic dysfunction in the $CD34^+$ or $CD34^-CD14^+$ cells. In a survey of cells from diabetic subjects, cultures of both $CD14^+$ cell containing $CD34^-$ PBMCs and $CD34^+$ PBMCs produced significantly fewer endothelial cell than did cultures from non-diabetic patients.[10, 21]

Exactly what the contribution of monocytes is relative to other blood-derived cells, and what physiological and molecular factors govern their differentiation and incorporation into the endothelium remain unclear. Certainly recent data suggest that VEGF, basic fibroblast growth factor, insulin-like growth factor -1, and oncostatin modulate endothelial cell precursor function, and new work in our laboratory indicates that erythropoietin, the angiopoietins, and transforming growth factor-β1 can also modulate their growth and/or differentiation, but much more work is needed in this area.[5, 18]

5. CONCLUSION

It is clear that blood-derived cells play a pivotal role in promoting neovascularization and remodeling in at least some physiological settings, probably both by releasing factors that promote vascular growth and by acting as endothelial cell precursors. Among the circulating endothelial cell precursors, there appear to be at least two distinct phenotypes. The first is related to hematopoietic stem cells, such as $CD34^+$ cells, and may represent the true endothelial cell stem cell. The second is related to monocytes and probably functions as a (non-self renewing) progenitor cell, capable of differentiating in to multiple phenotypes including dendritic cells, macrophages, and endothelial cell. This postulated stem-progenitor cell relationship between $CD34^+$ and $CD14^+$ cells has yet to be proven. Moreover, whether the two populations respond differentially to various stimuli is unknown. We will continue to work to answer these questions and to clarify the interrelationship between the two in the context of endothelial growth and repair.

6. REFERENCES

1. T. Asahara, C. Bauters, C. Pastore, M. Kearney, S. Rossow, S. Bunting, N. Ferrara, J. F. Symes, and J. M. Isner, Local delivery of vascular endothelial growth factor accelerates reendothelialization and attenuates intimal hyperplasia in balloon- injured rat carotid artery, *Circulation*, **91**, 2793-801. (1995).
2. T. Asahara, T. Murohara, A. Sullivan, M. Silver, R. van der Zee, T. Li, B. Witzenbichler, G. Schatteman, and J. M. Isner, Isolation of putative progenitor endothelial cells for angiogenesis, *Science*, **275**, 964-7 (1997).
3. J. R. Crosby, W. E. Kaminski, G. C. Schatteman, J. C. Martin, E. W. Raines, R. A. Seifert, and D. F. Bowen-Pope, Endothelial cells of hematopoietic origin make a significant contribution to adult blood vessel formation., *Circ Res*, **87**, 728-30 (2000).
4. B. Fernandez Pujol, F. C. Lucibello, U. M. Gehling, K. Lindemann, N. Weidner, M. L. Zuzarte, J. Adamkiewicz, H. P. Elsasser, R. Muller, and K. Havemann, Endothelial-like cells derived from human CD14 positive monocytes, *Differentiation*, **65**, 287-300 (2000).

5. B. Fernandez Pujol, F. C. Lucibello, M. Zuzarte, P. Lutjens, R. Muller, and K. Havemann, Dendritic cells derived from peripheral monocytes express endothelial markers and in the presence of angiogenic growth factors differentiate into endothelial-like cells, *Eur J Cell Biol*, **80**, 99-110. (2001).

6. U. M. Gehling, S. Ergun, U. Schumacher, C. Wagener, K. Pantel, M. Otte, G. Schuch, P. Schafhausen, T. Mende, N. Kilic, K. Kluge, B. Schafer, D. K. Hossfeld, and W. Fiedler, In vitro differentiation of endothelial cells from AC133-positive progenitor cells, *Blood*, **95**, 3106-12 (2000).

7. F. George, C. Brisson, P. Poncelet, J. C. Laurent, O. Massot, D. Arnoux, P. Ambrosi, C. Klein-Soyer, J. P. Cazenave, and J. Sampol, Rapid isolation of human endothelial cells from whole blood using S- Endo1 monoclonal antibody coupled to immuno-magnetic beads: demonstration of endothelial injury after angioplasty, *Thromb Haemost*, **67**, 147-53 (1992).

8. M. A. Goodell, K. Brose, G. Paradis, A. S. Conner, and R. C. Mulligan, Isolation and functional properties of murine hematopoietic stem cells that are replicating in vivo, *J Exp Med*, **183**, 1797-806 (1996).

9. M. B. Grant, W. S. May, S. Caballero, G. A. Brown, S. M. Guthrie, R. N. Mames, B. J. Byrne, T. Vaught, P. E. Spoerri, A. B. Peck, and E. W. Scott, Adult hematopoietic stem cells provide functional hemangioblast activity during retinal neovascularization, *Nat Med*, **8**, 607-12. (2002).

10. M. Harraz, C. Jiao, H. D. Hanlon, R. S. Hartley, and G. C. Schatteman, Cd34(-) blood-derived human endothelial cell progenitors, *Stem Cells*, **19**, 304-12 (2001).

11. W. C. Hueper, and M. A. Russell, Capillary-like formations in tissue culture of leukocytes, *Arch. Exp. Zellforsch.*, **12**, 407-424 (1932).

12. K. A. Jackson, S. M. Majka, H. Wang, J. Pocius, C. J. Hartley, M. W. Majesky, M. L. Entman, L. H. Michael, K. K. Hirschi, and M. A. Goodell, Regeneration of ischemic cardiac muscle and vascular endothelium by adult stem cells, *J Clin Invest*, **107**, 1395-402. (2001).

13. Y. Lin, D. J. Weisdorf, A. Solovey, and R. P. Hebbel, Origins of circulating endothelial cells and endothelial outgrowth from blood [see comments], *J Clin Invest*, **105**, 71-7 (2000).

14. J. R. Mackenzie, M. Hackett, C. Topuzlu, and D. J. Tibbs, Origin of arterial prosthesis lining from circulating blood cells, *Arch Surg*, **97**, 879-85 (1968).

15. Y. Noishiki, Y. Tomizawa, Y. Yamane, and A. Matsumoto, Autocrine angiogenic vascular prosthesis with bone marrow transplantation [see comments], *Nat Med*, **2**, 90-3 (1996).

16. R. C. Parker, The development of organized vessels in cultures of blood cells, *Science*, **77**, 544-46 (1933).

17. M. Peichev, A. J. Naiyer, D. Pereira, Z. Zhu, W. J. Lane, M. Williams, M. C. Oz, D. J. Hicklin, L. Witte, M. A. Moore, and S. Rafii, Expression of VEGFR-2 and AC133 by circulating human CD34(+) cells identifies a population of functional endothelial precursors, *Blood*, **95**, 952-8 (2000).

18. N. Quirici, D. Soligo, L. Caneva, F. Servida, P. Bossolasco, and G. L. Deliliers, Differentiation and expansion of endothelial cells from human bone marrow CD133(+) cells, *Br J Haematol*, **115**, 186-94. (2001).

19. R. Sbarbati, M. de Boer, M. Marzilli, M. Scarlattini, G. Rossi, and J. A. van Mourik, Immunologic detection of endothelial cells in human whole blood, *Blood*, **77**, 764-9 (1991).

20. J. Schaper, R. Konig, D. Franz, and W. Schaper, The endothelial surface of growing coronary collateral arteries. Intimal margination and diapedesis of monocytes. A combined SEM and TEM study, *Virchows Arch A Pathol Anat Histol*, **370**, 193-205. (1976).

21. G. C. Schatteman, H. D. Hanlon, C. Jiao, S. G. Dodds, and B. A. Christy, Blood-derived angioblasts accelerate blood-flow restoration in diabetic mice, *J Clin Invest*, **106**, 571-578 (2000).

22. A. Schmeisser, C. D. Garlichs, H. Zhang, S. Eskafi, C. Graffy, J. Ludwig, R. H. Strasser, and W. G. Daniel, Monocytes coexpress endothelial and macrophagocytic lineage markers and form cord-like structures in Matrigel under angiogenic conditions, *Cardiovasc Res*, **49**, 671-80. (2001).

23. D. Scholz, W. Ito, I. Fleming, E. Deindl, A. Sauer, M. Wiesnet, R. Busse, J. Schaper, and W. Schaper, Ultrastructure and molecular histology of rabbit hind-limb collateral artery growth (arteriogenesis), *Virchows Arch*, **436**, 257-70. (2000).

24. S. M. Scott, M. G. Barth, L. R. Gaddy, and E. T. Ahl, Jr., The role of circulating cells in the healing of vascular prostheses, *J Vasc Surg*, **19**, 585-93 (1994).

25. Q. Shi, S. Rafii, M. H. Wu, E. S. Wijelath, C. Yu, A. Ishida, Y. Fujita, S. Kothari, R. Mohle, L. R. Sauvage, M. A. Moore, R. F. Storb, and W. P. Hammond, Evidence for circulating bone marrow-derived endothelial cells, *Blood*, **92**, 362-7 (1998).

26. Q. Shi, M. H. Wu, N. Hayashida, A. R. Wechezak, A. W. Clowes, and L. R. Sauvage, Proof of fallout endothelialization of impervious Dacron grafts in the aorta and inferior vena cava of the dog, *J Vasc Surg*, **20**, 546-56; discussion 556-7 (1994).

27. H. Sinzinger, P. Fitscha, H. Kritz, W. Rogatti, and J. O. Grady, Prostaglandin E1 decreases circulating endothelial cells, *Prostaglandins*, **51**, 61-8 (1996).

28. M. M. Stump, J. L. Jordan, M. E. DeBakey, and B. Halpert, Endothelium grown from circulating blood on isolated intravascular Dacron hub, *Am J Pathol*, **43**, 361-7 (1963).

29. J. Waltenberger, J. Lange, and A. Kranz, Vascular endothelial growth factor-A-induced chemotaxis of monocytes is attenuated in patients with diabetes mellitus: A potential predictor for the individual capacity to develop collaterals, *Circulation*, **102**, 185-90 (2000).
30. G. C. White, and M. S. Parshley, Growth of in vitro blood vessels from bone marrow of adult chickens, *American Journal of Anatomy*, **89**, 321-345 (1950).
31. M. H. Wu, Q. Shi, A. R. Wechezak, A. W. Clowes, I. L. Gordon, and L. R. Sauvage, Definitive proof of endothelialization of a Dacron arterial prosthesis in a human being, *J Vasc Surg*, **21**, 862-7 (1995).

EVIDENCE FROM A LEUKEMIA MODEL FOR MAINTENANCE OF VASCULAR ENDOTHELIUM BY BONE-MARROW-DERIVED ENDOTHELIAL CELLS

Eberhard Gunsilius*

1. SUMMARY

The maintenance of tissues of virtually all organs depends on a sufficient blood supply. During embryogenesis, primitive blood vessels are formed de novo by the aggregation of angioblasts, a process that is termed *vasculogenesis*. In postnatal life, the development of new blood vessels is restricted to the female reproductive tract (during the ovulatory cycle) and to sites of wound healing, and occurs through a process called *angiogenesis*, i.e. the sprouting of new vessels from the preexisting vasculature.

However, neovascularization can also occur under pathological conditions, e.g. tumor cells can "switch on" angiogenesis. New blood vessels bring in nutrients and proteins, so the tumor mass can expand. In fact, neovascularization appears to be one of the crucial steps in the transition of a tumor from a small cluster of malignant cells to a visible macroscopic tumor capable of spreading to other organs via the vasculature throughout the body. The association of tumor growth with the development of a vascular network was recognized nearly a century ago.

Using a leukemia model, chronic myelogenous leukemia (CML), we were able to provide evidence for the existence of a hemangioblastic progenitor cell in the bone marrow of adult humans. Using the pathognomonic BCR-ABL-fusion gene as a genetic marker present in virtually all bone marrow derived cells of patients with CML, we were able to show that endothelial cells belong to the malignant cell clone, since they also contain the BCR-ABL-fusion gene. Our data suggest that CML arises from a hemangioblastic progenitor cell, the progeny of which are malignant blood cells and genotypically clonal endothelial cells. Thus, we provide substantial evidence that indeed a hemangioblast exists in the bone marrow of human adults.[1] In addition, our data imply that normal as well as genotypically malignant bone-marrow-derived endothelial cells can contribute to maintenance angiogenesis in the vascular endothelium, a condition that is consistent with postnatal vasculogenesis. These findings were recently confirmed by other groups and should help in elucidating the pathophysiology of malignant and

---

* Tumor-Biology & Angiogenesis Lab., Division of Hematology & Oncology, University Innsbruck, Austria. Email: eberhard.gunsilius@uibk.ac.at

Novel Angiogenic Mechanisms: Role of Circulating Progenitor Endothelial Cells.
Edited by Nicanor I. Moldovan, Kluwer Academic/Plenum Publishers, 2003.

nonmalignant disorders. The integration of bone-marrow-derived endothelial cells into the vascular endothelium has implications for the development of vascular targeting strategies (e.g., gene therapy) for vascular diseases, inflammatory disorders, and cancer. The characterization of the hemangioblast at a clonal level as well as the translation of these findings into a clinically applicable concept for the delivery of therapeutic genes to malignant tumors is currently in progress in our laboratory.

2. HEMATOPOIETIC PROGENITOR CELLS

All stem cells have the capability of self-renewal, i.e. they can continually reproduce themselves. Cells from the very earliest embryo (up to about the 16 cell stage) are totipotent stem cells. They are capable of forming all cells of the body, including the cells required to support embryonic and fetal development. More restricted stem cells (progenitor cells) also have the ability to self-renew, but their capacity to differentiate into various tissues seems to be limited, e.g. hematopoietic progenitor cells are thought to be limited in generating blood cells.

In adults, the production of blood cells of all types is accomplished by bone marrow derived progenitor cells. The amount of active bone marrow is known to be about 2,600 g, with approximately 1.26×10^{12} marrow cells. Alexander Maximow, working in St. Petersburg as a military doctor in 1909, was the first to suggest that there is a hematopoietic "stem" cell with the morphological appearance of a "lymphocyte" capable of migrating through the blood to microecological niches that would allow them to proliferate and differentiate along lineage specific pathways.[2]

Hematopoietic progenitor cells (HPC) are nowadays defined as clonogenic cells that can self renew and maintain multilineage hematopoiesis. Pluripotent HPC differentiate into oligolineage progenitor cells which loose their self-renewal capacity and themselves are giving rise to mature blood cells. Various committed progenitor cells giving rise to lymphoid or myeloid cells have been identified recently.[3,4] The generation of mature blood cells from pluripotent HPC involves a highly regulated progression through successive stages as commitment to a specific cell lineage, terminal differentiation of lineage restricted progenitor cells and growth arrest. A number of transcription factors and cytokines have been shown to influence the differentiation of hematopoietic cells and their lineage-restricted progeny.[5] During postnatal life HPC constitute a very small compartment, with estimates varying from less than 0.05% to up to 0.5% of cells in the bone marrow.

The surface phenotype of HPC is poorly defined. However, the presence of CD34[6], AC133[7] and the absence of CD38, HLA-DR and other lineage associated markers defines a cell population with the ability to restore hematopoiesis in recipients receiving myeloablative doses of chemoradiotherapy. Besides in bone marrow, such cells can also be found in umbilical cord blood and in very low number in peripheral blood. HPC can be "mobilized" from the bone marrow into the bloodstream by chemotherapy and/or hematopoietic cytokines such as G-CSF, GM-CSF, SCF and IL-3.[8]

Recently, the expression of KDR, a receptor for vascular endothelial growth factor became a tool for flow-cytometric analyses of very early hematopoietic progenitor cells, as seemingly only 5-10 KDR^+ cells ($CD34^+CD38^-KDR^+$) were necessary for restoring full hematopoiesis in lethally irradiated mice.[9]

3. HEMATOANGIOGENIC DEVELOPMENT IN THE EMBRYO

The embryo is thought to provide specific conditions for the emergence and expansion of hematopoietic stem cells. The yolk-sac was initially believed to be the unique organ providing hematopoietic progenitor cells that can colonize the embryo. It was thought that no other embryonic tissue has the potential to generate hematopoietic cells. During embryogenesis, nucleated red blood cells arise in the extraembryonic yolk sac and circulate through the embryo, thus providing oxygen to the embryonic tissues. However, in the avian embryo, also intraembryonic structures have been shown to initiate definitive hematopoiesis. This neighbors the dorsal aorta, and so the corresponding region of the mouse embryo was investigated. This region includes splanchnic mesoderm surrounding the entoderm of the developing gut and the endothelium of the developing blood vessels and was named paraaortic splanchnopleura (P-SP). In vitro analysis of the hematopoietic potential of P-SP as well as aorta-gonad-mesonephros (AGM) derived cells at the single cell level revealed that they were pluripotent, i.e. capable of generating blood cells of all lineages. Recently it was shown in mouse embryos that the intraembryonic splanchnopleura and the AGM gives rise to definitive multilineage hematopoiesis independent from the yolk-sac.[10]

Hematopoiesis in the embryo is closely associated with vasculogenesis. Vasculogenesis is the new formation of blood vessels from endothelial cells (in contrast to angiogenesis with names the generation of blood vessels through sprouting from preexisting vessels). Endothelial cells differentiate from the outer part of mesodermal cell clusters, whereas the inner cell mass generates blood cells.[11] A number of surface molecules is expressed on both, hematopoietic cells within blood islands and by endothelial cells lining the embryonic aorta, as CD34, TIE-2, CD31, CD45, VE-Cadherin and KDR2.

4. EVIDENCE FOR A HEMANGIOBLASTIC PROGENITOR CELL IN ADULT BONE MARROW

Wilhelm His, a histopathologist, performed extensive histological studies on embryonic development. He found blood islands and endothelial cells always close together during embryogenesis and thus he postulated a common precursor cell for hematopoietic cells and cells of the endothelial cell lineage.[12] Florence Sabin extended these studies and studied living embryos. She investigated chick embryos and suggested that angioblasts are derived from mesodermal cells and themselves are generating blood vessels and red blood cells.[13]

Fouad Shalaby from Toronto added in 1995 substantial evidence for the existence of a hemangioblastic progenitor cell. He generated knockout mice with a homozygous defect for flk-1, that is the VEGF-receptor-2. The offspring of those mice died in utero at day 9.5 post coitum due to a lack of blood islands *and* endothelial cells. Thus, VEGF and its receptor are essential for the development of blood vessels and blood cells, suggesting a common ancestor, at least during embryonic development.[14] Napoleone Ferrara and others added further evidence by the generation of knockout mice deficient for the gene encoding VEGF. They could show that even the lack of a single allele of this gene is embryonic lethal due to the lack of blood vessel formation and the absence of blood islands.[15,16]

Anne Eichmann has shown that KDR[+] cells sorted from early chick mesoderm, before vascularization, can generate hematopoietic cells and endothelial cells in vitro.[17] Choi and her co-workers cultured embryonic bodies (generated from mouse embryonic stem cells) in the presence of VEGF, kit-ligand and conditioned medium from an endothelial cell line. The embryonic bodies formed colonies of round immature cells (called blast-colony forming cells, BL-CFC) that expressed a number of genes shared by hematopoietic cells and endothelial cells, i.e. tal-1/SCL. They were able to show that under defined conditions, BL-CFC can generate hematopoietic cells as well as adherent cells with characteristics of endothelial cells.[18] This observations strongly suggest that the BL-CFC resemble cells with hemangioblastic properties.

In 1997, Takayuki Asahara from Jeff Isner's laboratory in Boston showed that endothelial cells can be generated from CD34/KDR positive blood cells of adult species.[19] Thus, we questioned whether we can use a leukemia model to elucidate if indeed a hemangioblastic precursor cell capable of generating both, blood cells and cells of the endothelial cell lineage, is present in the bone-marrow of adult humans. We choose chronic myelogenous leukemia (CML), a disease that is thought to derive from a pluripotent hematopoietic progenitor cell. CML, first described by Virchow in 1845,[20] is characterized by a unique chromosomal translocation, t(9;22)[21,22] (which is present in virtually all bone-marrow-derived immature and mature myelomonocytic cells as well as dendritic cells[23] and sometimes in T-lymphocytes.)[21] The molecular counterpart of the Philadelphia-chromosome is the BCR-ABL fusion gene.[24] After the transposition of genetic material between chromosomes 9 and 22, chromosome 22 is named "Philadelphia-Chromosome". A p[210] BCR-ABL fusion gene is produced by the fusion of the c-abl protooncogene (chromosone 9) and the abelson tyrosine kinase gene (abl, chromosome 22). Thus, if a common progenitor of hematopoietic cells and cells of the endothelial cell lineage exists in the adult bone marrow, endothelial cells grown from blood precursors of patients with CML should contain this BCR-ABL fusion gene as a clonal marker.

To test this hypothesis, we screened pluripotent hematopoietic progenitor cells, committed blood precursors, and endothelial cells which we generated in vitro from peripheral blood or bone marrow derived blood progenitor cells of patients with CML for the BCR-ABL fusion gene.

Six patients undergoing peripheral blood progenitor cells mobilization according to a phase-II protocol running at our institution[25] were choosen for this study. Mononuclear blood cells (enriched by density gradient centrifugation and depleted from monocytes/macrophages by repetitive plastic adherence) from peripheral blood, mobilized blood and/or bone-marrow were cultured at a density of approximately one million cells in fibronectin-coated 8-well chamber slides using a medium sufficient for the generation of endothelial cells.

A small proportion of the mononuclear cells became adherent within 2 hours of culture, and after 5 days clusters containing cells with cytological features of endothelial cells such as spindle shape and granularity were present. These expressed endothelial cell antigens (CD34[+], CD31[+], von Willebrand factor[+], P1H12/CD146[+], CD14[-]) showed binding of Ulex europeuus agglutinin-1, and incorporated acetylated LDL. After 10 days the endothelial-cell population accounted for more than 90% of the cultured cells, proliferated, became semiconfluent, formed tubes and networks in vitro and could be maintained in culture for several weeks.

When these cultured cells were analyzed for the presence of the BCR-ABL fusion gene by fluorescence in-situ hybridization, up to 56% of the cultured endothelial cells were found to contain the CML-specific translocation.

Thus, we provide evidence that cells of the endothelial lineage are part of the malignant cell clone in CML. Since FLK-1$^{-/-}$ mouse embryos (knockouts for the gene encoding the receptor for vascular endothelial growth factor-2) do not show vasculogenesis or develop blood islands, a common progenitor of endothelial cells and hemopoietic progenitor cells has been postulated.[14] Now, our observations provide formal evidence for the existence of this precursor cell with hemangioblastic features in human adults, in that both endothelial cells and pluripotent and committed hematopoietic progenitor cells contained the BCR-ABL fusion gene and therefore must have been arisen from a common ancestor. Thus, almost 100 years after its postulation,[12] it is apparent that a hemangioblast exists in the bone marrow of human adults.[1]

However, these data can be interpreted in several ways. Apart from the suggestion that CML may arise from a bipotent hemangioblast present in the adult is the possibility, especially in the light of the data suggesting that mature endothelial cells can yield blood cells, that perhaps mature hematopoietic cells can give rise to endothelial cells. Another possible interpretation is that CML may arise in a multipotent stem cell capable of giving rise to cell types other than blood and endothelium.

5. INTEGRATION OF BCR/ABL$^+$ ENDOTHELIAL CELLS INTO THE BLOOD VESSEL ENDOTHELIUM

Endothelial cells are among those exhibiting the lowest replication level in the body, with only 0.01% cells engaged in cell division at any time. But nevertheless, vascular endothelial cells that are going lost from the vessel intima through necrosis or apoptosis must be replaced (a process we call maintenance angiogenesis).

To investigate if bone marrow derived endothelial cells can contribute to maintenance angiogenesis in patients with CML, we used once more the clonal genetic marker which is present in virtually all bone-marrow derived cells of patients with CML and applied a BCR-ABL-specific gene probe to endothelial cells from the intimal layer of blood vessels in CML. Indeed, single BCR-ABL positive endothelial cells were found in myocardial blood vessels.[1]

This finding of BCR-ABL-expressing endothelial cells in the endothelium of myocardial blood vessels suggests that genotypically malignant endothelial cells can contribute to the vascular endothelium of patients with CML in vivo.

6. NORMAL BONE MARROW DERIVED ENDOTHELIAL CELLS CONTRIBUTE TO MAINTENANCE ANGIOGENESIS

We next investigated whether normal donor-type bone-marrow-derived endothelial cells are present in the vascular endothelium after allogeneic transplantation of hematopoietic stem cells (HSC). For this, a patient who received an HLA-mismatched HSC graft and subsequently died after transplantation was choosen. Donor-derived endothelial cells were detectable in the vascular endothelium of the recipient, as shown by the presence of donor HLA-antigens on the recipient's vascular endothelial cells.

Thus, we showed that in humans normal endothelial cells derived from the donor bone marrow can integrate into the recipient's vascular endothelium.

These data were recently corroborated by others. Crosby and colleagues transplanted bone-marrow from mice carrying a clonal marker into recipients and they were able to show that bone marrow derived endothelial cells (carrying the clonal marker) integrate into the blood vessel endothelium.[26] Moreover, their data suggest a role for postnatal vasculogenesis through the de novo formation of blood vessels through bone marrow derived endothelial cells, since they found up to 11% bone-marrow derived endothelial cells in vessels of granulation tissue.[27]

Emma Lagaij and her colleagues obtained renal biopsy samples from patients that had undergone renal transplantation. Using xy-FISH (for sex-mismatched transplants), monoclonal antibodies against ABO-antigens (for blood group mismatched transplants, endothelial cells express ABO-antigens), or antibodies against HLA-antigens (for HLA-mismatched transplants), they could show that indeed endothelial cells within the transplanted kidney are recipient derived. They also found a correlation between the amount of recipient derived endothelial cells in the graft and the rate of early and late graft-rejection.[28]

Gao et al. used a similar approach (xy-mismatch) to investigate the fate of endothelial cells in liver venules of human hepatic allografts. They also found a significant proportion of endothelial cells in liver venules to be of recipient origin. Moreover, using a mouse bone-marrow transplantation model, they were able to show that the endothelial cells that repopulate the liver venules are bone-marrow derived.[29] The group of Dr. Anversa has very recently shown in humans that after heart transplantation a significant proportion of the coronary endothelial cells express a recipient phenotype.[30]

7. TUMOR INDUCED VASCULOGENESIS?

The growth of malignant tumors is dependent on a sufficient blood supply. Moreover, for hematogenic spread, tumor cells must gain access to the blood vasculature to travel with the blood stream to distant organs. Vascular endothelial growth factor (VEGF) mediates both, the formation of new blood vessels by sprouting, intussusception or cooption of preexisting vessels, and is a potent inducer of vascular hyperpermeability.[31,32] An intriguing alternative to this established model of tumor induced neoangiogenesis is vasculogenesis, i.e. the new formation of blood vessels from bone marrow derived endothelial progenitor cells or angioblasts circulating in peripheral blood. Asahara and colleagues have described the generation of endothelial cells from blood derived progenitor cells.[19] They also showed in a mouse model that bone marrow derived endothelial cells can contribute to tumor vessel formation.[33] These findings are consistent with a role of postnatal vasculogenesis in tumor-induced blood vessel formation.

A prerequisite for tumor induced vasculogenesis is the secretion of soluble mediators from the malignant cells that are capable to induce mobilization of endothelial progenitor cells from the bone marrow. Indeed, it has been shown that granulocyte-macrophage colony stimulating factor (GM-CSF) and VEGF have the ability to increase the number of circulating EPC by mobilizing such cells from the bone marrow.[34,35] Since VEGF can be produced by colorectal cancer cells, the release of VEGF from colorectal tumors might be a mechanism to recruit EPC from the bone marrow for tumor-vasculogenesis and, moreover, to induce vascular permeability and thereby engaging the access of metastatic tumor cells to the bloodstream. Supporting this concept, we found substantially elevated plasma levels of VEGF in tumor draining veins of patients with colorectal cancer in vivo.[36]

Currently, we are using transgenic animals to elucidate the amount of bone-marrow derived endothelial cells to the tumor vasculature. We have gained evidence for the selective homing of ex-vivo generated endothelial cells or their precursors into tumors (unpublished data). When ex-vivo generated, fluorochrome-labeled EC/EPC were injected systemically into animals bearing a (stereotactically implanted) orthotopic brain tumor, the labelled cells were found closely associated with tumor vessels or integrated into the tumor vessel endothelium. Next, the mechanism(s) how these cells are homing into tumor vessels will be investigated by the selective silencing of adhesion-molecule encoding genes.

8. REFERENCES

1. Gunsilius, E., Duba, H. C., Petzer, A. L., Kähler, C. M., Grünewald, K., Stockhammer, G., Gabl, C., Dirnhofer, S., Clausen, J., and Gastl, G.: Evidence from a leukaemia model for the maintenance of the blood vascular endothelium by bone-marrow derived endothelial cells. Lancet 355:1688-1691 (2000).
2. Maximow, A.: Der Lymphozyt als gemeinsame Stammzelle der verschiedenen Blutelemente in der embryonalen Entwicklung und im postfetalen Leben der Säugetiere. Folia Haematologica VIIII 8:125-134 (1909).
3. Akashi, K., Traver, D., Miyamoto, T., and Weissman, I. L.: A clonogenic common myeloid progenitor that gives rise to all myeloid lineages [In Process Citation]. Nature 2000.Mar.9;404(6774):193-7. 404:193-197 (2000).
4. Kondo, M., Weissman, I. L., and Akashi, K.: Identification of clonogenic common lymphoid progenitors in mouse bone marrow. Cell 91:661-672 (1997).
5. Alexander, W. S.: Cytokines in hematopoiesis. Int.Rev.Immunol. 16:651-682 (1998).
6. Berenson, R. J., Andrews, R. G., Bensinger, W. I., Kalamasz, D., Knitter, G., Buckner, C. D., and Bernstein, I. D.: Antigen CD34+ marrow cells engraft lethally irradiated baboons. J.Clin.Invest 81.951-955 (1988).
7. Yin, A. H., Miraglia, S., Zanjani, E. D., Almeida-Porada, G., Ogawa, M., Leary, A. G., Olweus, J., Kearney, J., and Buck, D. W.: AC133, a novel marker for human hematopoietic stem and progenitor cells. Blood 90:5002-5012 (1997).
8. Duhrsen, U., Villeval, J. L., Boyd, J., Kannourakis, G., Morstyn, G., and Metcalf, D.: Effects of recombinant human granulocyte colony-stimulating factor on hematopoietic progenitor cells in cancer patients. Blood 72:2074-2081 (1988).
9. Ziegler, B. L., Valtieri, M., Porada, G. A., De Maria, R., Muller, R., Masella, B., Gabbianelli, M., Casella, I., Pelosi, E., Bock, T., Zanjani, E. D., and Peschle, C.: KDR receptor: a key marker defining hematopoietic stem cells. Science 285:1553-1558 (1999).
10. Cumano, A., Dieterlen-Lievre, F., and Godin, I.: Lymphoid potential, probed before circulation in mouse, is restricted to caudal intraembryonic splanchnopleura. Cell 86:907-916 (1996).
11. Flamme, I. and Risau, W.: Induction of vasculogenesis and hematopoiesis in vitro. Development 116:435-439 (1992).
12. His, W.: Lecithoblast und Angioblast der Wirbelthiere. Abhandl KS Ges Wiss Math Phys 22:171-328 (1901).
13. Sabin, F. R.: Preliminary note on the differentiation of angioblasts and the method by which they produce blood-vessels, blood-plasma and red blood cells as seen in the living chick. Anatomical Record 13:199-204 (1917).
14. Shalaby, F., Rossant, J., Yamaguchi, T. P., Gertsenstein, M., Wu, X. F., Breitman, M. L., and Schuh, A. C.: Failure of blood-island formation and vasculogenesis in Flk-1- deficient mice. Nature 376:62-66 (1995).
15. Ferrara, N., Carver-Moore, K., Chen, H., Dowd, M., Lu, L., O'Shea, K. S., Powell-Braxton, L., Hillan, K. J., and Moore, M. W.: Heterozygous embryonic lethality induced by targeted inactivation of the VEGF gene. Nature 380:439-442 (1996).
16. Carmeliet, P., Ferreira, V., Breier, G., Pollefeyt, S., Kieckens, L., Gertsenstein, M., Fahrig, M., Vandenhoeck, A., Harpal, K., Eberhardt, C., Declercq, C., Pawling, J., Moons, L., Collen, D., Risau, W.,

and Nagy, A.: Abnormal blood vessel development and lethality in embryos lacking a single VEGF allele. Nature 380:435-439 (1996).

17. Eichmann, A., Corbel, C., Nataf, V., Vaigot, P., Breant, C., and Le Douarin, N. M.: Ligand-dependent development of the endothelial and hemopoietic lineages from embryonic mesodermal cells expressing vascular endothelial growth factor receptor 2. Proc.Natl.Acad.Sci.U.S.A 94:5141-5146 (1997).

18. Choi, K., Kennedy, M., Kazarov, A., Papadimitriou, J. C., and Keller, G.: A common precursor for hematopoietic and endothelial cells. Development 125:725-732 (1998).

19. Asahara, T., Murohara, T., Sullivan, A., Silver, M., van der Zee, R., Li, T., Witzenbichler, B., Schatteman, G., and Isner, J. M.: Isolation of putative progenitor endothelial cells for angiogenesis. Science 275:964-967 (1997).

20. Virchow, R.: Weisses Blut. Neue Notizen aus dem Gebiet der Natur-und Heilkunde. Florieps Neue Notizen 36:151. (1845).

21. Nowell, P. C. and Hungerford, D. A.: A minute chromosome in human granulocytic leukemia. Science 132:1497-1501 (1960).

22. Rowley, J. D.: Letter: A new consistent chromosomal abnormality in chronic myelogenous leukaemia identified by quinacrine fluorescence and Giemsa staining. Nature 243:290-293 (1973).

23. Eibl, B., Ebner, S., Duba, C., Bock, G., Romani, N., Erdel, M., Gachter, A., Niederwieser, D., and Schuler, G.: Dendritic cells generated from blood precursors of chronic myelogenous leukemia patients carry the Philadelphia translocation and can induce a CML-specific primary cytotoxic T- cell response. Genes Chromosomes.Cancer 20:215-223 (1997).

24. Groffen, J., Stephenson, J. R., Heisterkamp, N., de Klein, A., Bartram, C. R., and Grosveld, G.: Philadelphia chromosomal breakpoints are clustered within a limited region, bcr, on chromosome 22. Cell 36:93-99 (1984).

25. Petzer, A., Hochenburger, E, Haun, M., Duba, C., Grünewald, K., Hoflehner, E., Sill, H, Linkesch, W, Gastl, G, and Gunsilius, E.: High-dose hydroxyurea plus G-CSF mobilizes bcr-abl negative progenitor cells (CFC, LTC-IC) into the blood of newly diagnosed CML-patients at any time of hematopoietic regeneration. J.Hematother.Stem Cell Res. 11: 293-300 (2002).

26. Crosby, J. R., Kaminski, W. E., Schatteman, G., Martin, P. J., Raines, E. W., Seifert, R. A., and Bowen-Pope, D. F.: Endothelial cells of hematopoietic origin make a significant contribution to adult blood vessel formation. Circ.Res. 87:728-730 (2000).

27. Pinedo, H. M., Verheul, H. M., D'Amato, R. J., and Folkman, J.: Involvement of platelets in tumour angiogenesis? Lancet 352:1775-1777 (1998).

28. Lagaaji, E. L., Cramer-Knijnenburg, G. F., van Kemenade, F. J., van Es, L. A., Brujin, J. A., and van Krieken, J. H. J. M.: Endothelial cell chimerism after renal transplantation and vascular rejection. Lancet 357:33-37 (2001).

29. Gao, Z., McAlister, V. C., and Williams, G. M.: Repopulation of liver endothelium by bone-marrow-derived cells. Lancet 357:932-933 (2001).

30. Quaini, F., Urbanek, K., Beltrami, A. P., Finato, N., Beltrami, C. A., Nadal-Ginard, B., Kajstura, J., Leri, A., and Anversa, P.: Chimerism of the transplanted heart. N.Engl.J.Med. 346:5-15 (2002).

31. Carmeliet, P.: Mechanisms of angiogenesis and arteriogenesis. Nat.Med. 6:389-395 (2000).

32. Carmeliet, P. and Jain, R. K.: Angiogenesis in cancer and other diseases. Nature 407:249-257 (2000).

33. Asahara, T., Masuda, H., Takahashi, T., Kalka, C., Pastore, C., Silver, M., Kearne, M., Magner, M., and Isner, J. M.: Bone marrow origin of endothelial progenitor cells responsible for postnatal vasculogenesis in physiological and pathological neovascularization. Circ.Res. 85:221-228 (1999).

34. Asahara, T., Takahashi, T., Masuda, H., Kalka, C., Chen, D., Iwaguro, H., Inai, Y., Silver, M., and Isner, J. M.: VEGF contributes to postnatal neovascularization by mobilizing bone marrow-derived endothelial progenitor cells. EMBO J. 18:3964-3972 (1999).

35. Takahashi, T., Kalka, C., Masuda, H., Chen, D., Silver, M., Kearney, M., Magner, M., Isner, J. M., and Asahara, T.: Ischemia- and cytokine-induced mobilization of bone marrow-derived endothelial progenitor cells for neovascularization. Nat.Med. 5:434-438 (1999).

36. Gunsilius, E, Tschmelitsch, J., Eberwein, M., Schwelberger, H., Spizzo, G., Kähler, C. M., Stockhammer, G., Lang, A., and Gastl, G.: In-vivo release of vascular endothelial growth factor from colorectal carcinomas. Oncology 62(4):313-7 (2002).

CROSS TALK BETWEEN HAEMATOPOIESIS AND ANGIOGENESIS

Domenico Ribatti°, Angelo Vacca*, Beatrice Nico°, Enrico Crivellato**, Giuseppe De Falco*, and Marco Presta^

1. EARLY DEVELOPMENT OF THE ENDOTHELIAL AND HAEMATOPOIETIC LINEAGES IS CLOSELY LINKED

The relationship between endothelial cells (EC) and haematopoietic cells (HC) has been seen as an indication that a common progenitor, the haemangioblast, gives rise to both cell types in the yolk sac, the initial site of haematopoiesis and of blood vessel formation (Murray, 1934). Generation of haemangioblasts take place from embryonic stem cells (ESC) or from yolk sac blood islands or from intraembryonic AGM (aorta-gonad-mesonephros) region, containing the dorsal aorta, genital ridge/gonads and pro-mesonephros.

The existance of the haemangioblast has been inferred from the expression of a number of genes in developing HC and EC. Its role as a common progenitor is primarily deduced from the transient formation of "blast colonies" giving rise to both lineages in differentiating ESC cultures (Choi et al., 1998). The detection of similar colonies in dissected mouse embryo cultures indicates that haemangioblasts may be formed *in vivo* (Palis et al., 2001).

Upon appropiate cytokine stimulation, haemangioblasts differentiate into angioblasts that, in turn, differentiate into endothelium, which then form capillaries. Haemangioblasts also generate haematopoietic SC, which, in turn, generate common lymphocytes progenitors that differentiate into T, B and natural killer cells, and common myeloid progenitors that differentiate to erythroid, granulocyte-macrophage and megakaryocytic progenitors.

°Department of Human Anatomy and Histology, *Department of Biomedical Sciences and Human Oncology, University of Bari Medical School, Policlinico, I-70124 Bari, Italy* *Department of Medical and Morphological Researches, Section of Anatomy, University of Udine Medical School, I-33100; Udine, Italy; ^Unit of General Pathology and Immunology, Department of Biomedical Sciences and Biotechnology, University of Brescia Medical School, I-25123, Brescia, Italy.

Novel Angiogenic Mechanisms: Role of Circulating Progenitor Endothelial Cells.
Edited by Nicanor I. Moldovan, Kluwer Academic/Plenum Publishers, 2003.

It has been suggested that haematopoiesis and angiogenesis are two apparently independent processes (Ribatti et al., 2000). In fact, it has been demonstrated that several haematopoietic cytokines and interleukins (IL), such as granulocyte-colony stimulating factor (G-CSF), granulocyte macrophage-colony stimulating factor (GM-CSF), erythropoietin (Epo), interleukin 3 (IL-3), IL-4, IL-6 and IL-8, affect several functions of endothelial cells and that, in turn, angiogenic cytokines, such as fibroblast growth factor-2 (FGF-2) and vascular endothelial growth factor (VEGF) affect several functions of haematopoietic cells.

2. ANGIOGENIC POTENTIAL OF RECOMBINANT HUMAN EPO (RHEPO) AND GM-CSF

We have demonstrated that rhEpo induces a pro-angiogenic phenotype in human endothelial cell (Ribatti et al., 1999). This phenotype included both early, such as increase in cell proliferation and matrix metalloproteinase-2 (MMP-2) production, and late angiogenic events, such as, differentiation into vascular tubes when endothelial cells are seeded on Matrigel. Moreover, endothelial cells expressed EpoR that bound to JAK-2 and that induced its transient activation after Epo exposure. In the CAM assay the angiogenic activity of rhEpo was similar to that exerted by FGF-2 (Figure 1). Finally, endothelial cells of the CAM expressed Epo receptor that colocalizes with factor VIII von Willebrand factor (FVIII-vWF) related antigen. Taken together, these data demonstrated that rhEpo acts as a direct angiogenic factor.

More recently, we have also shown that GM-CSF *in vivo* induces angiogenesis and activates JAK-2 and signal transducers and activators of transcription (Valdembri et al., 2002). This cytokine had an angiogenic activity in the CAM without recruitment of inflammatory cells and induces vessel sprouting from chicken aorta rings. When added to CAM, subnanomolar concentrations of GM-CSF caused a rapid phosphorylation in tyrosine residues of JAK-2 persisting at least for 10 min. Furthermore, we have shown that signal transducers and activators of transcription such as STAT-3, but not STAT-5, also were phosphorylated for 30 min after GM-CSF stimulation. AG-490, a JAK-2 inhibitor, reduced in a dose-dependent manner the angiogenic effect of GM-CSF in the CAM. These findings provide the first evidence that JAK-2/STAT-3 pathway is activated *in vivo* and partecipates in vessel formation triggered by GM-CSF.

3. THE DEVELOPMENT OF A NEW PARADIGM: THE IMPORTANCE OF ANGIOGENESIS IN THE HEAMATOLOGICAL MALIGNANCIES

Angiogenesis and the production of angiogenic factors are fundamental for tumor progression in the form of growth, invasion and metastasis (Folkman, 1995). Tumor angiogenesis is linked to a switch in the equilibrium between positive and negative regulators (Hanahan and Folkman, 1996). In normal tissues, vascular quiescence is maintained by the dominant influence of endogenous angiogenesis inhibitors over angiogenic stimuli. Tumor angiogenesis, on the other hand, is induced by increased secretion of angiogenic factors and/or downregulation of angiogenesis inhibitors.

Solid tumour growth consists of an avascular and a subsequent vascular phase. Assuming that it is dependent on angiogenesis and that this depends on the release of

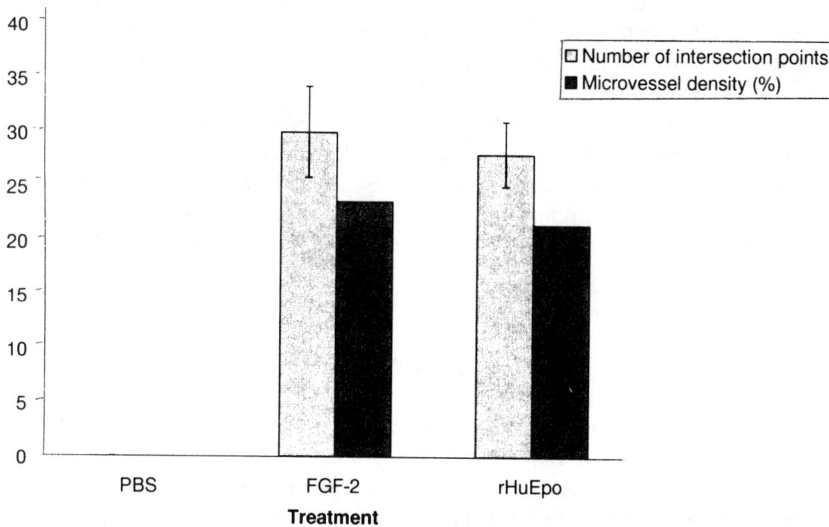

Figure 1. Angiogenesis by recombinant human erythropoietin. Quantitation of the angiogenic response in the CAM assay. The response was assessed histologically by a planimetric method of 'point counting' at day 12 of incubation, as described in Ribatti et al., (1999).

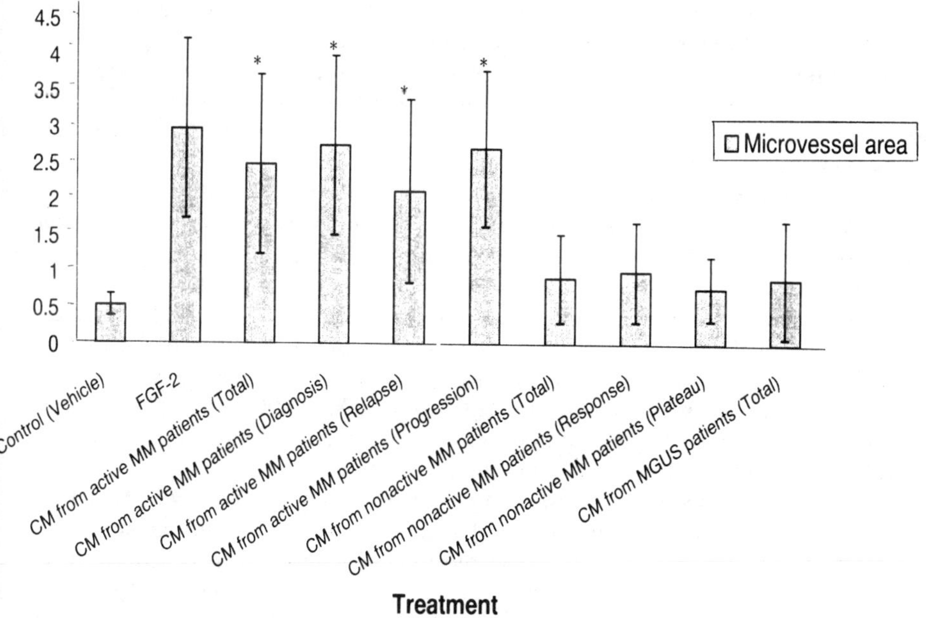

Figure 2. Angiogenesis in multiple myeloma. Quantitation of the angiogenic response of the plasma cell conditioned media in the CAM assay (01 vs. Nonactive MM patients).

angiogenic factors, acquisition of angiogenic capability can be seen as an expression of progression from neoplastic transformation to tumor growth and metastasis (Folkman, 1990). Practically all solid tumors, including tumors of the colon, lung, breast, cervix, bladder, prostate and pancreas, progress through these phases.

While it is well established that the growth of solid tumors is angiogenesis-dependent, it was still assumed that haematological malignancies were not. The role of angiogenesis in growth and survival of these tumors has only recently been realized. Since 1994, it has been demonstrated that the progression of several haematopoietic cancers is clearly related to their degree of angiogenesis (Bertolini et al., 2000; Mangi et al., 2000).

4. ANGIOGENESIS IN MULTIPLE MYELOMA (MM)

In 1994 we published a paper where we observed that in MM there is a significant correlation between the extent of bone marrow angiogenesis and disease progression (Vacca et al., 1994). We investigated the microvessel area density of bone marrow in patients with active MM and compared it with that of patients with inactive MM and with that of patients with monoclonal gammopathies of undetermined significance (MGUS) and we showed that the microvessel area was significantly different when active and non-active disease were compared.

As the progression from *in situ* to invasive and metastatic solid tumors is accompanied and enhanced by the switch from the prevascular to the vascular phase (Hanahan and Folkman, 1996), these findings suggest that active MM may represent the 'vascular phase' of plasma cell tumors, and non active MM and benign lesions their 'prevascular phase'. Moreover, since bone marrow angiogenesis and labelling index % (LI %) are closely associated with the phases of MM activity and are mutually correlated, and since LI% is a prognostic factor, it may well that the MGUS and non-active MM are at risk of progression towards the larger mass steady-state (active MM), if the bone marrow shows angiogenesis.

In 1999 we published a further study concerning angiogenesis in MM (Vacca et al., 1999). In this study, we used endothelial cells to evaluate their response to the plasma cell conditioned media (CM). The stimulation to endothelial cell migration induced by CM of active MM was stronger as compared to that of non active MM and benign lesions. The monocyte chemotaxis stimulation test was performed in a similar manner, and the CM of patients with active MM gave results similar to those described for endothelial cell chemotaxis. To stimulate angiogenesis *in vivo*, we used the CAM implanted with gelatin sponges loaded with the CM. The CM of 80% active MM patients induced an angiogenic response. By contrast, only 30% and 20% of CM from non active MM and MGUS patients, respecitively, induced the response (Figure 2).

We obtained by means of the ELISA assay evidence in favour of FGF-2 production by MM plasma cells during the active phase. The levels were significantly higher in the lysate of active MM patients compared with those of non active MM. Based on these findings, we wondered whether FGF-2 was actually involved in the *in vitro* induction of endothelial cell angiogenic phenotype and CAM angiogenesis by the plasma cell CM. An assessment was made of the effects of neutralizing anti-FGF-2 antibody on the CM samples from active MM patients that induced both endothelial cell and monocyte functions *in vitro* and angiogenesis *in vivo* in the CAM assay. The antibody was able to inhibit all these functions.

5. ANGIOGENESIS IN B-CELL NON-HODGKIN'S LYMPHOMAS (B-NHL)

We found in B-NHL a significantly higher microvessel counts in high-grade lymphomas than in low-grade lymphomas, implying that angiogenesis occuring in B-NHL increases with tumor progression (Ribatti et al., 1996). Moreover, the stroma of B-NHL reacted intensely with both basement membrane components, namely laminin and type IV collagen, whose linear co-expression was significantly associated with low-grade and follicular intermediate-grade B-NHL, whereas expression of laminin alone in a granular pattern was detected in diffuse intermediate-grade and high-grade tumors. Finally, ultrastructural analysis showed immature vessels characterized by a slit-like lumen, more frequently in high grade B-NHL.

6. ROLE OF MMP IN ANGIOGENESIS IN HAEMATOLOGICAL MALIGNANCIES

MMPs production *in vivo* and *in vitro* is increased in reponse to angiogenic agents (Coussens and Werb, 1996). In some conditions, such as diabetic retinopathy, proteinase involvement may be confined to angiogenesis (Folkman, 1995); in others, such as cancer (Johnson et al., 1998) proteinase activity is thought to be an integral part of both generalized tissue remodeling and angiogenesis.

We studied the production of MMP-2 and –9 in lymphoblastoid cell lines such as Burkitt's lymphoma, B-cell lymphoblastic leukemia, T-cell lymphoblastic leukemia and MM (U 266) cell lines (Vacca et al., 1998). All cell lines were found to secrete the different forms of the MMPs.

We further focused on the invasive potential of bone marrow plasma cells during MM progression (Vacca et al., 1999). We found that plasma cells of MGUS and MM patients secreted MMP-2 and -9 by gelatin zymography and that plasma cells of MGUS and MM patients expressed the MMP-2 and -9 mRNA, as evaluated by *in situ* hybridization. The MMP-2 secretion and mRNA related signal was stronger in patients with active MM than in those with non active MM and with MGUS. The MMP-9 secretion and mRNA related signal was lower than that of MMP-2 in all patient groups and overlapped between the groups.

Given the ability of MMP-2 to degrade the major components of the interstitial stroma and subendothelial basement membrane, these findings suggest that plasma cells of active MM patients are especially capable of invading both the stroma and the basement membrane.

7. ROLE OF STROMAL COMPARTMENT IN ANGIOGENESIS IN HAEMATOLOGICAL MALIGNANCIES

The majority of studies in neoplastic transformation have focused attention on events that occur within transformed cells. Recent works have addressed the microenvironment of tumor cells and documented its importance in supporting tumor progression (Park et al., 2000). Host inflammatory cells, including lymphocytes, macrophages and mast cells, may act synergistically with tumor cells by secreting the same or other angiogenic factors, as occurs.

Mast cells (MC) play a pivotal role in this synergism (Ribatti et al., 2001). MC density is highly correlated with the extent of both normal and pathological angiogenesis, such as that in chronic inflammatory diseases and tumors. MC release a variety of factors known to enhance angiogenesis, namely heparin, histamine and tryptase, a variety of cytokines, such as transforming growth factor-β, tumor necrosis factor-α, interleukin-8, FGF-2 and VEGF implicated in angiogenesis.

In this context, we studied patients with active and nonactive MM and MGUS for MC counts in relation to the FVIII-vWF microvessel area in their bone marrow (Ribatti et al., 1999). Results showed that the MC counts were significantly higher in active MM patients than in non active MM (Figure 3). At the ultrastructural level, MC with semilunar aspect and piecemeal partial degranulation of their granules were a frequent finding in active MM. The MC morphology, unlike the IgE-mediated massive degranulation which occurs during the immediate hypersensitivity reactions, implies slow degranulation that takes place in chronic inflammation and in solid tumors, and suggests chronic and progressive stimulation of MC degranulation.

This study led to hypothesize that MC are recruited and activated in the bone marrow by MM plasma cells and that angiogenesis that occurs in MM is mediated, at least in part, by angiogenic factors (FGF-2, VEGF, tryptase) contained in their secretory granules.

We have further also investigated about the role of MC in tumor angiogenesis in B-NHL and we demonstrated that angiogenesis was correlated with the total metachromatic (Figure 4) and MC tryptase-positive counts, and that both counts increased in step with the increase in malignancy grades (Ribatti et al., 1998; 2000).

More recently, we have shown also in bone marrow samples of patients with myelodysplastic syndromes a high correlation between microvessel counts and both total and metachromatic and tryptase reactive MC and that both parameters increase simultaneously with tumor progression (Ribatti et al., 2002).

Overall, our data agree with those showing a close relationship between mast cell density and angiogenesis during tumor progression.

8. ANTI-ANGIOGENESIS IN HAEMATOLOGICAL MALIGNANCIES

Anti-angiogenesis was proposed as a cancer therapy over 20 years ago by Judah Folkman in an editorial (Folkman, 1971). The term 'anti-angiogenesis' was introduced to describe treatment designed to prevent the induction of new blood vessels and perhaps reduce the number of those already present. Inhibitors of angiogenesis are grouped as class 1 (specific and semi-specific) and class 2 (non-specific), depending on whether they only inhibit proliferation and/or migration of endothelial cells or are also cytotoxic for tumor cells. The list of compounds reported to possess anti-angiogenic activity is extensive. Anti-angiogenic therapy is applicable to a wide variety of solid tumors and there is evidence that tumors do not develop resistance to its effects is most likely because the low mutagenic potential of endothelial cells (Talks and Harris, 2000).

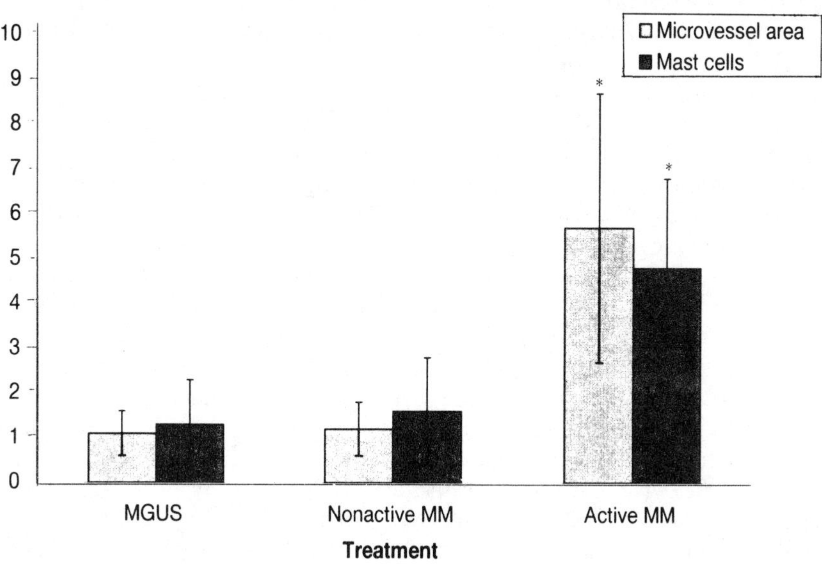

Figure 3. Microvessel area and mast cell counts in the bone marrow of patients with multiple myeloma. The microvessel area is expressed in μm^2 (001 vs. Nonactive MM and MGUS).

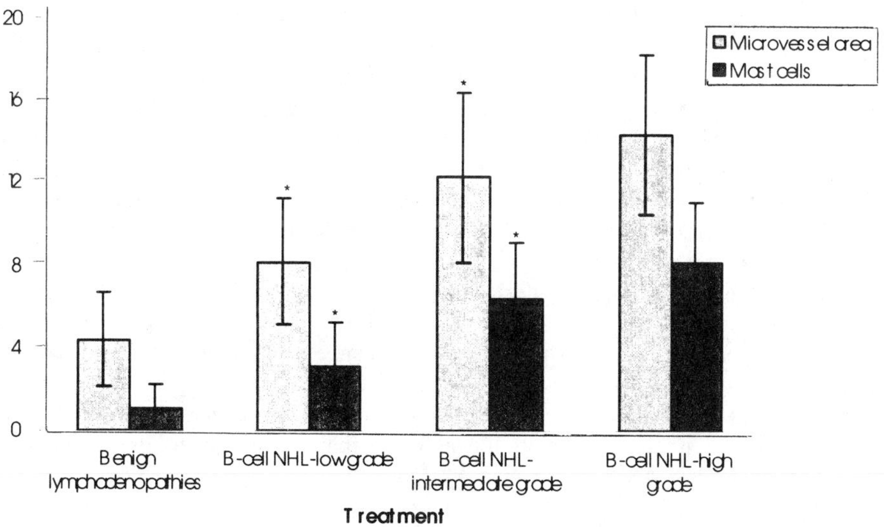

Figure 4. Microvessel area and mast cell counts in the bone marrow of patients with B-cell non-Hodgkin's lymphoma. The microvessel area is expressed in μm^2 (05 vs. the preceding group).

Conventional cytotoxic chemoterapeutic drugs have been used at low and non-cytotoxic concentrations as anti-angiogenic. Anti-endothelial effects have been demonstrated *in vitro* and *in vivo* for several cytostatic agents. The presence of dividing endothelial cells in newly forming tumor blood vessels should render such vessels - in contrast to the mature vessels found in normal adult tissues - sensitive to the cytotoxic effects of such drugs.

In this context, we have studied the effects of vinblastine (VBL) on endothelial cells functions involved in angiogenesis, namely proliferation, chemotaxis, spreading on fibronectin, secretion of MMP-2 and -9, and morphogenesis on Matrigel, whereas its effects on angiogenesis were studied *in vivo* by using the CAM assay (Vacca et al., 1999). *In vitro* at non-cytotoxic doses (0.1-0.25, 0.5, 0.75 and 1 pmol/L) VBL impacted all these functions. *In vivo* in the CAM assay, at the same doses, VBL displayed a dose-dependent anti-angiogenic activity, and it inhibited the angiogenic response induced in the same assay by FGF-2 (Figures 5, 6). These results suggest that VBL has an antiangiogenic activity at very low, noncytotoxic doses, and that anti-angiogenesis by VBL could be used to treat a wide spectrum of angiogenesis-dependent diseases.

We also demonstrated that the taxanes paclitaxel and its analog docetaxel inhibited endothelial proliferation, chemotaxis and morphogenesis *in vitro* and angiogenesis *in vivo* (Vacca et al., 2002). These anti-angiogenic effets were directly dose-dependent and obtained at docetaxel 0-5-1 nM and 2-4 nM paclitaxel and were accompanied by a progressive, though moderate increase of apoptotic cells in proportion to the dose. Inhibition of these *in vitro* endothelial functions is in close agreement with inhibition of *in vivo* angiogenesis in the CAM assay (Figure 7).

Finally, we demonstrated that the purine analog 6-methylmercaptopurine riboside (6-MMPR) modulated the angiogenic activity of FGF-2 *in vitro* and affect blood vessel formation *in vivo* in the CAM assay (Figure 8) (Presta et al., 1999). In contrast, 6-methylmercaptopurine, 2-aminopurine, and adenine were devoid of anti-angiogenic activity, thus indicating that subtle structural differences may determine the ability of purine analogs to affect neovascularization. On this basis, we addressed the possibility that 6 thioguanine (6-TG) may act as an anti-angiogenic molecule, this activity contributing to its efficacy in acute myelogeneous leukemia (AML) therapy.

6-TG was evaluated for the capacity to affect various steps of the angiogenic process (i.e. cell proliferation, motility, endothelial cell sprouting, collagen invasion, and formation of capillary-like structures) induced by FGF-2 and/or VEGF in cultured endothelial cells of different origin (Presta et al., 2002). The *in vitro* observations were compared to the effect of 6-TG on *in vivo* neovascularization in the CAM assay under basal condition or during neovascularization induced by FGF-2 or VEGF or by human leukemia LIK cells grafted onto the CAM. Finally, we evaluated bone marrow neovascularization in AML patients given maintenance therapy with 6-TG. The results demonstrated that 6-TG inhibited different steps of the angiogenic process *in vitro* and exerted a potent anti-angiogenic activity in the CAM. Moreover, its anti-angiogenic capacity together with its antimetabolite activity, may contribute to its action during maintenance therapy in AML.

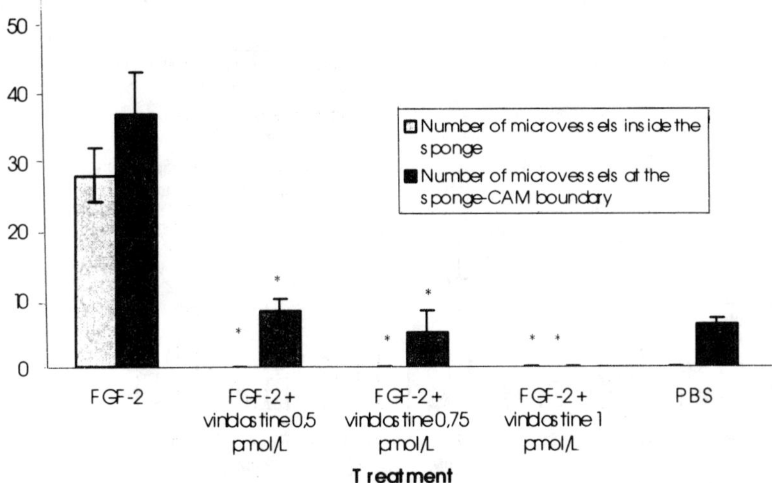

Figure 5. Anti-angiogenesis by vinblastine. Macroscopic quantitation of the vascular density in the CAM assay was assessed as the number of vessels at 50 x at the sponge-CAM boundary (01 for the within-sample comparison - Wilcoxon-Wilcox Test).

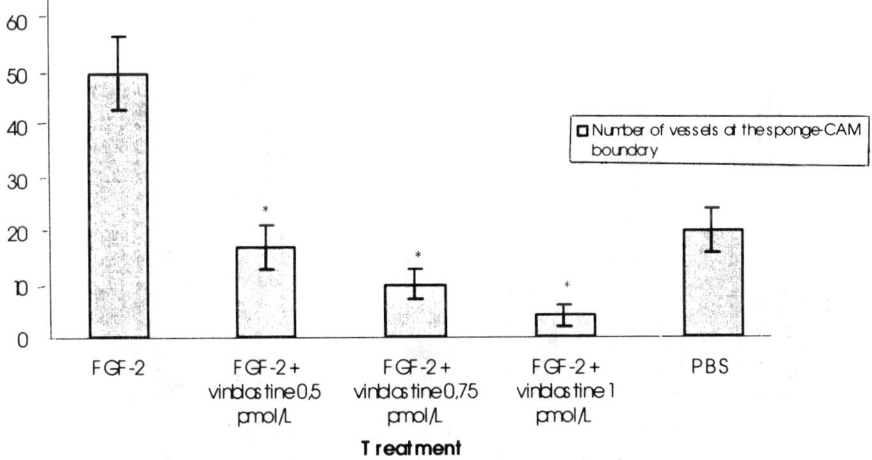

Figure 6. Anti-angiogenesis by vinblastine. Microscopic quantitation of the vascular density in the CAM assay at the sponge-CAM boundary and inside the sponge (01 for the within-sample comparison - Wilcoxon-Wilcox Test).

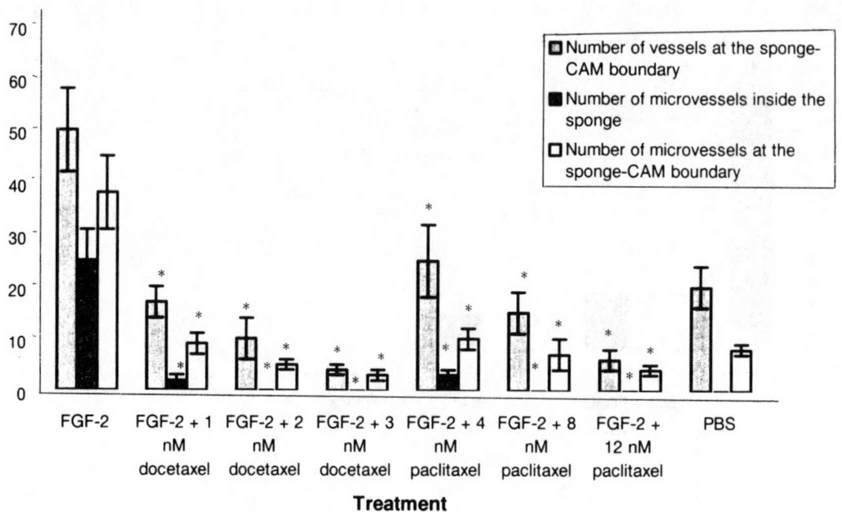

Figure 7. Anti-angiogenesis by docetaxel and paclitaxel. Macroscopic and microscopic assessment of vascular density in the CAM assay (01 for the within-sample comparison - Wilcoxon-Wilcox Test).

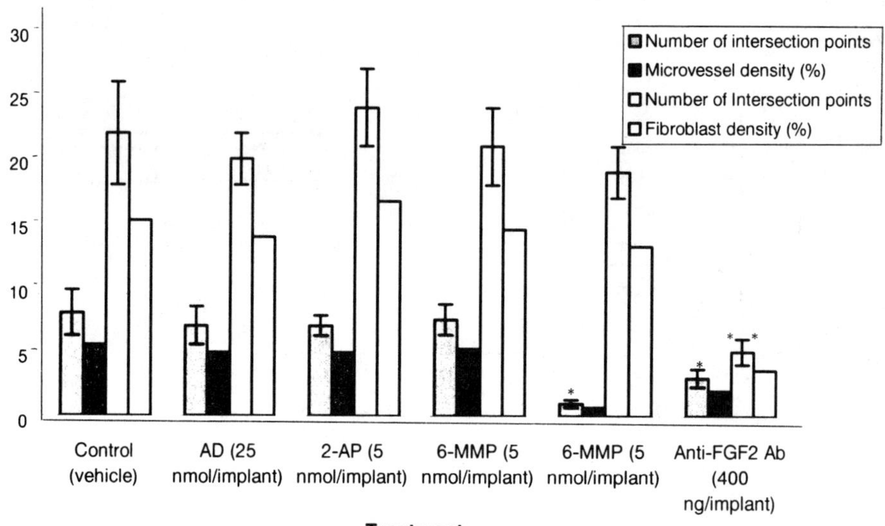

Figure 8. Anti-angiogenesis by purine analogues. Quantitation of the angiogenic response in the CAM assay (001 vs. Control , AD, 2-AP and 6-MMP **p < 0.001 vs. all other groups).

The use of low doses in "metronomic" chemotherapy (namely, very frequent or continuous low-dose chemotherapy) as anti-angiogenic targeting strategy seems particularly effective against drug-resistant tumors, especially whent it is combined with a second anti-angiogenic drug (Fidler and Ellis, 2000; Kerbel, 2000).

While it is premature to establish whether anti-angiogenesis will be of benefit in haematological malignancies, developing treatment strategies that target both the stromal and tumor compartments, such as combining traditional cytotoxic chemotherapy with anti-angiogenic agents, may indeed have an impact on drug resistance and improve the therapeutic response in these diseases.

9. ACKNOWLEDGEMENTS

This work was supported in part by a grant from Fondazione Italiana per la Lotta al Neuroblastoma, Genoa, Italy, to DR, and by a grant from Associazione Italiana per la Ricerca sul Cancro (AIRC), Milan, Italy, to AV and MP.

10. REFERENCES

Bertolini, F., Mancuso, P., Gobbi, A., and Pruneri, G., 2000. The thin red line: angiogenesis in normal and malignant hematopoiesis. *Exp. Hematol.* **28**: 993-1000.

Choi, K., Kennedy, M., Kazarov, A., Papadimitriou, J.C., and Keller, G., 1998. A common precursor for hematopoietic and endothelial cells. *Development* **125**: 725-732.

Coussens, L.M., and Werb, Z., 1996. Matrix metalloproteinases and the development of cancer. *Chemic. Biol.* **3**: 895-904.

Fidler, I.J., and Ellis, L.M., 2000. Chemotherapeutic drugs – more really is not better. *Nature Med.* **6**: 500-502.

Folkman, J., 1971. Tumor angiogenesis: therapeutic implications. *New Engl. J. Med.* **285**: 1182-1186.

Folkman, J., 1990. What is the evidence that tumors are angiogenesis dependent? *J. Natl. Cancer Inst.* **22**: 4-6.

Folkman, J., 1995. Clinical applications of research in angiogenesis. *N. Engl. J. Med.* **333**: 1757-1763.

Hanahan, D., and Folkman, J., 1996. Patterns and emerging mechanisms of the angiogenic switch during tumorigenesis. *Cell* **86**: 353-364.

Johnson, L.L:, Dyer, R., and Hupe, D.J., 1998. Matrix metalloproteinases. *Curr. Opin. Chem. Biol.* **4**: 466-471.

Kerbel, R.S., 2000. Tumor angiogenesis: past, present and the near future. *Carcinogenesis* **21**: 505-515.

Mangi, M.H., and Newland, A.C., 2000. Angiogenesis and angiogenic mediators in haematological malignancies. *Br. J. Haematol.* **111**: 43-51.

Murray, P.D.F., 1934. The development *in vitro* of blood of the chick embryo. *Proc. R. Soc. B* **111**: 497-524.

Palis, J., Chan, R.J., Koniski, A., Patel, R., Starr, M., and Yoder, M.C., 2001. Spatial and temporal emergence of high proliferative potential haematopoietic precursors during murine embryogenesis. *Proc. Natl. Acad. Sci. USA* **98**: 4528-4533.

Park, C.C., Bissell, M.J., and Barcellos-Hoff, M.H., 2000. The influence of the microenvironment on the malignant phenotype. *Mol. Med. Today* **6**: 324-329.

Presta, M., Rusnati, M., Belleri, M., Morbidelli, L., Ziche, M., and Ribatti, D., 1999. Purine analogue 6-methylmercaptopurine riboside inhibits early and late phases of the angiogenic process. *Cancer Res.* **59**: 2417-2424.

Presta, M., Belleri, M., Vacca, A., and Ribatti, D., 2002. Anti-angiogenic activity of the purine analog 6-thioguanine. *Leukemia*, in press.

Ribatti, D., Vacca, A., Nico, B., Fanelli, M., Roncali, L., and Dammacco, F., 1996. Angiogenesis spectrum in the stroma of B-cell non-Hodgkin's lymphomas. An immunihistochemical and ultrastructural study. *Eur. J. Haematol.* **56**: 45-53.

Ribatti, D., Nico, B., Vacca, A., Marzullo, A., Calvi, N., Roncali, L., and Dammacco, F., 1998. Do mast cells help to induce angiogenesis in B-cell non Hodgkin's lymphomas? *Br. J. Cancer* **77**: 1900-1906.

Ribatti, D., Presta, M., Vacca, A., Ria, R., Giuliani, R., Dell'Era, P., Nico, B., Roncali, L., and Dammacco, F., 1999. Human erythropoietin induces a pro-angiogenic phenotype in cultured endothelial cells and stimulates neovascularization *in vivo Blood* **93**: 2627-2636.

Ribatti, D., Vacca, A., Roncali, L., and Dammacco, F., 2000. Hematopoiesis and angiogenesis: a link between two apparently independent processes, *J. Hematother. Stem Cell Res.* **9**: 13-19.

Ribatti, D., Vacca, A., Marzullo, A., Nico, B., Ria, R., Roncali, L., and Dammacco, F., 2000. Angiogenesis and mast cell density with tryptase activity increase simultaneously with pathological progression in B-cell non-Hodgkin's lymphomas. *Int. J. Cancer* **85**: 171-185.

Ribatti, D., Vacca, A., Nico. B., Crivellato, E., Roncali, L., and Dammacco, F., 2001. The role of mast cells in tumour angiogenesis. *Br. J. Haematol.* **115**: 514-521.

Ribatti, D., Polimeno, G., Vacca, A., Marzullo, A., Crivellato, E., Nico, B., Lucarelli, G., and Dammacco, F., 2002. Correlation of bone marrow angiogenesis and mast cells with tryptase activity in myelodysplastic syndromes. *Leukemia*, in press

Talks, K.L., and Harris, A.L., 2000. Current status of antiangiogenic factors. *Br. J. Haematol.* **109**: 477-489.

Vacca. A., Ribatti, D., Roncali, L., Serio, G., Silvestris, F., and Dammacco, F., 1994. Bone marrow angiogenesis and progression in multiple myeloma. *Br. J. Haematol.* **87**: 503-508.

Vacca, A., Ribatti, D., Iurlaro, M., Albini, A., Minischetti, M., Bussolino, F., Pellegrino, A., Ria, R., Rusnati, M., Presta, M., Vincenti, V., Persico, M.G., and Dammacco, F., 1998. Human lymphoblastoid cells produce extracellular matrix-degrading enzymes and induce endothelial cell proliferation, migration, morphogenesis and angiogenesis. *Int. J. Clin. Lab. Res.* **28**: 55-68.

Vacca, A., Ribatti, D., Presta, M., Minischetti, M., Iurlaro, M., Ria, R., Albini, A., Bussolino, F., and Dammacco, F., 1999. Bone marrow neovascularization, plasma cell angiogenic potential and matrix metalloproteinase-2 secretion parallel progression of human multiple myeloma. *Blood* **93**: 3064-3073.

Vacca, A., Iurlaro, M., Ribatti, D., Minischetti, M., Nico, B., Ria, R., Pellegrino, A., and Dammacco, F., 1999. Antiangiogenesis is produced by nontoxic doses od vinblastine. *Blood* **94**: 4143-4155.

Vacca, A., Ribati, D., Iurlaro, M., Merchionne, F., Nico, B., Ria, R., and Dammacco, F., 2002. Docetaxel versus paclitaxel for antiangiogenesis. *J. Hematother. Stem Cell Res.* **11**: 103-118.

Valdembri, D., Serini, G., Vacca, A., Ribatti, D., and Bussolino, F., 2002. *In vivo* activation of JAK-2/STAT-3 pathway during angiogenesis induced by GM-CSF. *FASEB J.* **16**: 225-227.

THE CONTRIBUTION OF ADULT HEMATOPOIETIC STEM CELLS TO RETINAL NEOVASCULARIZATION

Maria B. Grant, Sergio Caballero, Gary A. J. Brown, Steven M. Guthrie, Robert N. Mames, Timothy Vaught, and Edward W. Scott*

1. INTRODUCTION

Retinal neovascular diseases such as diabetic retinopathy and retinopathy of prematurity are among the leading causes of vision impairment throughout the world. Retinal neovascularization is thought to occur in response to a hypoxic insult, which leads to changes in the existing microvasculature such as pericyte death and subsequent endothelial cell proliferation.[1, 2] Compensatory neovascularization then results in the formation of aberrant and pathologic capillaries. An important question whose answer would have broad implications for potential therapeutic strategies is the origin of the cells responsible for compensatory neovascularization.

Postnatal neovascularization has been attributed to angiogenesis, a process characterized by sprouting of new capillaries from pre-existing blood vessels.[3] Recent evidence by Asahara and coworkers has demonstrated the presence of circulating endothelial progenitor cells (EPC) that may be recruited to areas of neovascularization.[4] EPCs that are capable of contributing to *in vitro* capillary formation can be derived from bone marrow cells.[5-8] Angiogenic growth factors such as vascular endothelial growth factor (VEGF)[4, 9] and granulocyte/macrophage colony stimulating factor (GM-CSF)[10] can promote the release of these cells from the bone marrow into the circulation, and promote new blood vessel formation.

Vasculogenesis is the process within the developing embryo whereby pluripotent progenitor cells are generated that are capable of contributing to the formation of blood and blood vessels.[11-14] These pluripotent stem cells are termed hemangioblasts. Hemangioblasts can also be produced from embryonic stem cells during *in vitro* differentiation in response to vascular endothelial growth factor.[11] However, definitive evidence for the existence of the hemangioblast within the adult bone marrow, and in particular for a functional role of such BM-derived cells in neovascularization, has been lacking until now.

* MBG, SC, GAJB, SMG, TV, EWS, University of Florida, Gainesville, FL, 32610.
  RNM, The Retina Center, Gainesville, FL, 32605.

Novel Angiogenic Mechanisms: Role of Circulating Progenitor Endothelial Cells.
Edited by Nicanor I. Moldovan, Kluwer Academic/Plenum Publishers, 2003.

2. ENDOTHELIAL CELL DERIVATION

Numerous studies support the contribution by EPC to blood vessel formation in the adult.[4, 9, 15, 16] However, since these studies are based on short-term transplant and acute injury models, it is not clear whether the cell type giving rise to circulating EPCs is a true hematopoietic stem cell (HSC) or some other progenitor such as the mesenchymal stem cell (MSC).

HSCs derived from adult bone marrow are classically defined by their ability to self renew while functionally repopulating the cells of the blood and lymph for the life of an individual,[17] as shown in schematic form in Figure 1. These abilities make HSCs clinically useful in therapeutic bone marrow transplantation for a variety of bone marrow diseases, including leukemia and lymphoma. HSCs can be highly enriched and quantified.[18] As with other tissue-derived stem cells, HSCs are thought to retain a high capacity for "plasticity" that would allow for the potential contribution of regenerative progenitors to non-hematopoietic tissues following injury or stress.[19, 20]

Circulating EPCs may be derived from MSCs or, potentially, from HSCs with hemangioblast properties. Current EPC enrichment procedures have failed to distinguish convincingly the origin of circulating EPC. Previous studies utilized acute injuries and described the incorporation of bone marrow-derived cells into newly formed vessels.

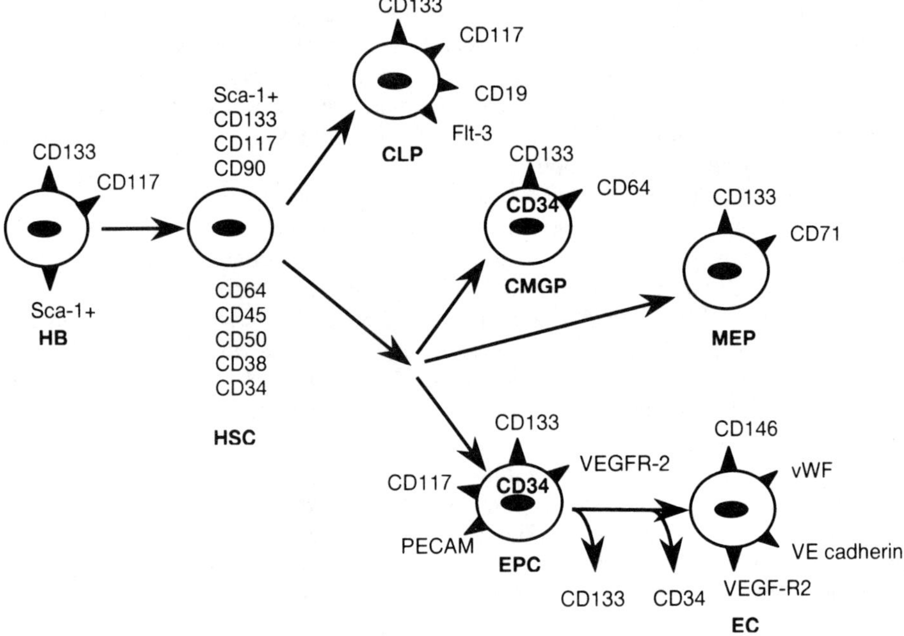

Figure 1. Schematic representation of potential endothelial cell lineage. Triangles represent surface antigens (as labeled) associated with each stage of differentiation. The proposed adult hemangioblast (HB) may give rise to the pluripotent hematopoietic stem cell (HSC), or may in fact be the same cell. HSCs give rise to common lymphocyte precursors (CLP), common monocyte/granulocyte precursors (CMGP), and megakaryocyte/erythrocyte precursors (MEP). One differentiation pathway results in endothelial progenitor cells (EPC), which may be recruited via the circulation to form mature endothelial cells (EC).

However, by the very design of these acute injury models, both the MSC and the HSC may contribute to the formation of new blood vessels. If the injury occurs long after bone marrow reconstitution, the MSC no longer remains in the bone marrow and only the HSC remains to participate in "regenerative" neovascularization. The ultimate origin of cells contributing to a regenerative process can only be confirmed by using a single-cell transplant approach.

Krause and coworkers accomplished full and durable reconstitution of a lethally irradiated mouse with a single BM-derived HSC then identified donor cells in multiple tissues such as the brain, heart, skeletal muscle, liver, and endothelium.[20] These results suggest the possibility of functional regeneration of multiple tissues by HSC-derived progenitors. In other transplant models hematopoietic progenitors have been shown to repopulate hepatocytes in the parenchymal liver to restore liver function following chemically induced injury,[21, 22] and to regenerate myocardium to improve cardiac function following infarction.[23]

Given these lines of evidence we hypothesized that the adult HSC is sufficiently plastic to act as a functional hemangioblast (e.g. form all blood cells and blood vessels) in an adult animal with retinal ischemia. To test this hypothesis a model of retinal neovascularization that mirrors the pathology seen in proliferative diabetic retinopathy was developed.[24] Using this novel murine model, we examined whether the adult HSC could provide functional hemangioblast activity in an adult animal after an ischemic challenge to the retina.

3. EXPERIMENTAL EVIDENCE FOR THE INVOLVEMENT OF HSC IN RETINAL NEOVASCULARIZATION

The availability of transgenic mice stably expressing green fluorescent protein (gfp) provided an important tool for exploring adult HSC plasticity. By transplanting bone marrow from these gfp⁺ transgenic animals into irradiated recipients, the resultant chimeras could be used in disease models. The presence of fully differentiated tissues expressing gfp in these chimeras would be evidence of bone marrow-derived stem cell transdifferentiation. Furthermore, gfp⁺ donor marrow was enriched for specific cell populations prior to transplanting into recipients. This provided a means for distinguishing the contribution of specific cell populations to the model being tested.

A consensus opinion exists that the diabetic milieu consists of a pro-thrombotic hematological state with increased levels of coagulant proteins, hyper-aggregable platelets, and poorly deformable red blood cells, all of which can lead to areas of capillary non-perfusion and resultant ischemia. Hypoxic damage to the microvasculature downstream of microthrombi may ultimately lead to the development of abnormal collateral vessels to compensate for the ischemic injury.

Unfortunately, the adult models of diabetes do not exhibit consistent and reproducible neovascularization. We therefore developed a new model of retinal angiogenesis utilizing the mouse eye and incorporating a combination of site-specific growth factor expression followed by photocoagulation-induced ischemia. The combination of these stimuli resulted in consistent and reproducible vascular engorgement, tortuosity, and development of neovascular tufts. By subjecting the aforementioned gfp chimeric mice to this model, the presence of gfp-expressing cells in the vasculature illustrated that bone marrow-derived stem cells could contribute to the development of new vessels.

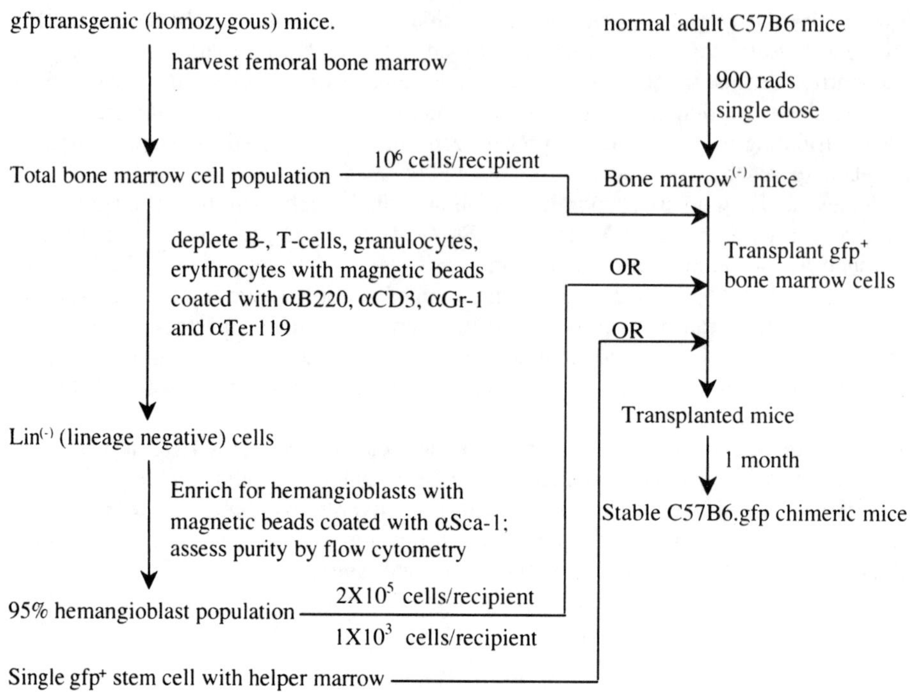

Figure 2. This flow chart depicts the process involved in generating the three types of C57B6.gfp chimeras used to examine stem cell contributions to retinal neovascularization. In the first type, whole bone marrow from gfp transgenic mice was used. In the second type, primary and secondary reconstitution was accomplished using a purified (Lin$^-$/Sca-1$^+$) HSC population. Finally, single HSCs were isolated and mixed with HSC-depleted helper marrow for single-cell reconstitution.

3.1. Chimeric Animals With gfp$^+$ Bone Marrow

The donor gfp transgenic strain was obtained from The Jackson Laboratory, Bar Harbor, ME. The strain carries gfp, driven by chicken beta-actin promoter and CMV intermediate early enhancer, in all of its cell types. Chimeric mice, referred to as C57B6.gfp, were generated by irradiating recipient C57BL/6J mice with 950 rads followed by intravenous injection of gfp$^+$ donor tissue. Three types of chimeras were used for these studies: those transplanted with whole bone marrow, those reconstituted with purified HSCs, and those reconstituted with a single donor HSC (Figure 2).

In order to purify the HSC compartment, harvested marrow was made into a single cell suspension and plated onto treated plastic dishes. Non-adherent cells were collected and subjected to three rounds of lineage antibody depletion (B220, CD3, CD4, CD8, CD11b, Gr-1, TER 119) until a small aliquot stained with PE-conjugated lineage Ab cocktail showed >95% lineage negative by flow cytometry. The Lin$^-$ cells were then positively selected for Sca-1 for 2-3 rounds until an aliquot showed greater than 95% Sca-1$^+$, Lin$^-$ purity. The Sca-1$^+$, Lin$^-$ cells were then stained for CD45 to confirm hematopoietic origin. For single HSC transplants Sca-1$^+$, c-kit$^+$, Lin$^-$ HSCs were first enriched by FACS sorting, and then individual HSCs were selected with micromanipulators via fluorescent microscopy. Individual gfp$^+$ HSCs were then mixed with 2 x 10^5 non-gfp$^+$ bone marrow cells that had been depleted of Sca-1$^+$ cells by magnetic beads prior to transplant into irradiated hosts.

3.2 Induction of Neovascularization

After durable hematopoietic reconstitution was established, chimeric mice were injected intravitreally with recombinant AAV expressing the full-length human VEGF gene under control of the CMV promoter. Four weeks after injection, the animals underwent laser photocoagulation of the vasculature with the purpose of creating occlusions and resultant ischemia. The beam from an Argon Green laser system at a wavelength 488-514 nm was applied to selected venous sites one disc area away from the optic nerve. Three weeks later the animals were killed, perfused with 4% buffered formaldehyde containing rhodamine-conjugated dextran, enucleated, and the retinas removed and mounted flat to evaluate neovascular development by fluorescence microscopy. Selected animals were perfused instead with Hoechst stain, enucleated, and the eyes cryosectioned for immunocytochemistry. The eyes from selected non-perfused animals were used for histochemistry.

3.3 Results

Figure 3 encapsulates the results obtained with the model system described herein. Injured eyes displayed pathologies consistent with ischemia-induced retinal neovascularization as seen in diseases such as diabetic retinopathy. These pathologies included vascular engorgement and tortuosity, and pre-retinal neovascularization (Figure 3A). In chimeric mice, the uninjured eyes showed circulating, bone marrow-derived gfp$^+$ cells, but few if any such cells exterior to the vessels (Figure 3B). By contrast, the injured eyes of chimeric animals evinced extensive areas of neovascularization comprised of gfp$^+$ cells forming entire vascular networks (Figure 3C). Staining sections from such eyes with endothelial cell marker such as PECAM-1 (Figure 3D-F), von Willebrand factor, or the pan-endothelial cell marker MECA32 (the latter two not shown) confirms that these cells were indeed endothelial cells.

All of the mice transplanted with highly enriched HSCs contained numerous new vessels observable in all quadrants of the retina. In every field examined in these retinas, at least two new areas of neovascularization were observed. This indicated that most injuries were repaired, in part, with donor-derived (i.e. gfp$^+$) cells. In contrast, mice that were reconstituted with whole bone marrow demonstrated qualitatively fewer gfp$^+$ cells in areas of neovascularization. Thus, the higher the number of HSCs used to reconstitute the chimeras, the greater the number of donor-derived endothelial cells were observed in neovascular areas. All of the chimeras, however, demonstrated functional hemangioblast activity – as defined by re-population of the blood and regeneration of blood vessels – that co-enriches with the HSC.

Durable, long-term reconstitution of the hematopoietic system in irradiated hosts is the classic definitive assay for HSC function. We performed secondary transplants of highly purified HSCs derived from primary recipients to confirm that the incorporation of gfp$^+$ endothelial cells in neovascular areas resulted from the self-renewing long-term re-

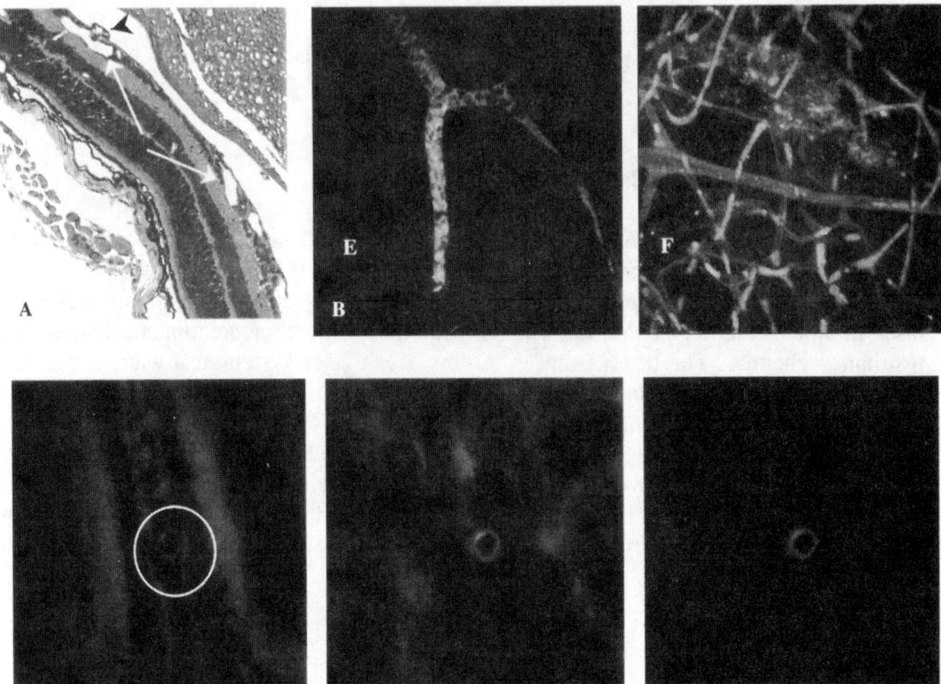

Figure 3. Panel A depicts a hematoxylin and eosin-stained section of an injured eye showing intraretinal vascular engorgement (arrows) and pre-retinal neovascularization (arrowhead) resulting from local VEGF overexpression followed by photocoagulation-induced ischemic injury. Panel B demonstrates the presence of gfp-expressing cells in the retinal circulation of the uninjured eye from a C57B6.gfp chimeric mouse. Note the absence of gfp$^+$ cells outside of the vessels. Panel C shows extensive formation of new vessels in the injured eye from the same animal as in Panel B. Preexisting vasculature appears red as a result of rho-damine-dextran perfusion. New vessels appear as either green only (un-perfused) tubes, or as yellow tubes resulting from the combined spectra of gfp and rhodamine. Panels D through F are the identical section of an injured eye from a serially reconstituted chimeric mouse that was perfused with Hoechst stain. The blue fluorescent Hoechst stain delineates a vessel in cross-section (circled in Panel D) that can be seen to express gfp (Panel E). The section was reacted with phycoerythrin-conjugated antibody to PECAM-1 (CD31) to detect endothelial cells. As can be seen in Panel F, the gfp$^+$ cells surrounding the lumen of the vessel are indeed endothelial cells as they express PECAM-1. For a color representation of this figure, see color insert at the end of book.

populating HSCs. All of the secondary reconstituted animals showed extensive gfp expression in retinal vasculature undergoing neovascular induction. Thus, a serially transplantable, multiple hematopoietic lineage-reconstituting adult HSC clearly has hemangioblast properties and can regenerate functional vasculature.

Finally, in order to confirm the HSC as the source of hemangioblast activity, we performed single HSC transplants using purified HSC from serially reconstituted chimeric animals. Individual gfp$^+$ HSCs were isolated manually and transplanted along with Sca-1-depleted, non-gfp bone marrow. The depleted marrow served as a source of short-term hematopoietic progenitors to enhance single HSC engraftment. In all animals that survived this procedure we observed robust gfp$^+$ endothelial cell contribution to new retinal vessel formation in the neovascular induction model. Thus, a single adult HSC can function as a hemangioblast.

4. DISCUSSION

In addition to the classic mechanisms for recruiting resident endothelial cells for compensatory angiogenesis, a potential role for circulating endothelial precursor cells is gaining acceptance.[5, 10, 25, 26] Our findings demonstrated that retinal neovascularization results not only from stimulation of local endothelial cells through an angiogenic process, but also relies on recruitment of undifferentiated precursor cells to aid in new blood vessel formation.

Circulating EPC may be derived from either MSCs or potentially from HSCs with hemangioblast properties. Traditional EPC enrichment procedures have failed to distinguish convincingly the origin of circulating EPC. We directly addressed this question by establishing both secondary transplant and single HSC transplant recipients that had durable reconstitution of their hematopoietic lineages. Reconstitution of secondary lethally irradiated hosts with enriched bone marrow-derived HSCs from primary transplants demonstrated the ability of HSCs to expand and self-renew, thus satisfying the definition of a stem cell.[17, 27] Serial transplantation also precludes MSC participation in the reconstitution because there is no evidence to indicate that MSCs are able to serially engraft.[28-31]

Adult stem cell transdifferentiation encompasses three facets: the ability to result in functional differentiated activity; the ability to self-renew; and clonality. Our model satisfied all of these requirements. Firstly, hemangioblast activity increased with the purity of HSCs. If the bone marrow-derived gfp$^+$ cells incorporated into new blood vessels were derived from MSCs, less neovascularization would be expected in mice undergoing transplantation with an enriched HSC population, as opposed to transplantation with whole bone marrow. Instead, the opposite was observed, indicating that HSC are major contributors to the functional vessel formation that occurs during neovascularization in the retina. Secondly, all previous models examining endothelial progenitor cells were short-term transplant models. These models could not clearly distinguish contributions from short term hematopoietic progenitors from HSCs, or HSCs from MSCs. Others have demonstrated that in bone marrow transplant recipients all MSCs were of recipient origin, with no donor MSC detectable.[28-32] The ability of the HSCs to reconstitute long-term multilineage hematopoiesis in a series of recipient animals has classically defined the HSC compartment. Using this model we demonstrated that the self-renewing adult HSCs compartment could also provide hemangioblast function. With the serial transplants it is still conceivable that different HSC clones contribute to blood versus blood vessel formation. The single HSC transplants formally demonstrated the clonal nature of adult HSC hemangioblast activity. The combination of these two approaches definitively proves that adult HSCs function as hemangioblasts.

To optimize the treatment of pathological neovascularization, the cellular source of the new blood vessels must be determined. Current treatment modalities focus on changing the local retinal milieu by photocoagulation. However, if the predominant cell responsible for neovascularization is derived from the bone marrow (as opposed to fully differentiated resident cells), then an entirely different therapeutic approach may be indicated.

5. ACKNOWLEDGEMENTS

The authors would like to thank Dr. Margaret I. Davis for her insights into and assistance in the immunocytochemistry of whole retinas. The work described was supported in part by grants from the Juvenile Diabetes Foundation (JDF 4-2000-847) and the National Eye Institute (EY012601 and EY007739) to MBG, and by the National Cancer Institute (CA72769) and the National Institute of Diabetes and Digestive and Kidney Diseases (DK52558) to EWS.

6. REFERENCES

1. M.B. Grant, B. Russell, C. Fitzgerald, and T. J. Merimee, Insulin-like growth factors in vitreous: studies in control and diabetic subjects with neovascularization, *Diabetes* **35** (4), 416 (1986).
2. G. A. Limb, A. H. Chignell, W. Green, F. LeRoy, and D. C. Dumonde, Distribution of TNF alpha and its reactive vascular adhesion molecules in fibrovascular membranes of proliferative diabetic retinopathy, *Br J Ophthalmol* **80** (2), 168 (1996).
3. J. Folkman and Y. Shing, Angiogenesis, *J Biol Chem* **267** (16), 10931 (1992).
4. T. Asahara, T. Takahashi, H. Masuda, C. Kalka, D. Chen, H. Iwaguro, Y. Inai, M. Silver, and J. M. Isner, VEGF contributes to postnatal neovascularization by mobilizing bone marrow-derived endothelial progenitor cells, *Embo J* **18** (14), 3964 (1999).
5. T Asahara, T Murohara, A Sullivan, M Silver, R van der Zee, and T Li, Isolation of putative progenitor endothelial cells for angiogenesis, *Science* **275**, 964 (1997).
6. U. M. Gehling, S. Ergun, U. Schumacher, C. Wagener, K. Pantel, M. Otte, G. Schuch, P. Schafhausen, T. Mende, N. Kilic, K. Kluge, B. Schafer, D. K. Hossfeld, and W. Fiedler, In vitro differentiation of endothelial cells from AC133-positive progenitor cells, *Blood* **95** (10), 3106 (2000).
7. V. Bhattacharya, P. A. McSweeney, Q. Shi, B. Bruno, A. Ishida, R. Nash, R. F. Storb, L. R. Sauvage, W. P. Hammond, and M. H. Wu, Enhanced endothelialization and microvessel formation in polyester grafts seeded with CD34(+) bone marrow cells, *Blood* **95** (2), 581 (2000).
8. Y. Lin, D. J. Weisdorf, A. Solovey, and R. P. Hebbel, Origins of circulating endothelial cells and endothelial outgrowth from blood, *J Clin Invest* **105** (1), 71 (2000).
9. C. Kalka, H. Masuda, T. Takahashi, R. Gordon, O. Tepper, E. Gravereaux, A. Pieczek, H. Iwaguro, S. I. Hayashi, J. M. Isner, and T. Asahara, Vascular endothelial growth factor(165) gene transfer augments circulating endothelial progenitor cells in human subjects, *Circ Res* **86** (12), 1198 (2000).
10. T. Takahashi, C. Kalka, H. Masuda, D. Chen, M. Silver, M. Kearney, M. Magner, J. M. Isner, and T. Asahara, Ischemia- and cytokine-induced mobilization of bone marrow-derived endothelial progenitor cells for neovascularization, *Nat Med* **5** (4), 434 (1999).
11. K. Choi, Hemangioblast development and regulation, *Biochem Cell Biol* **76** (6), 947 (1998).
12. D. M. Noden, Embryonic origins and assembly of blood vessels, *Am Rev Respir Dis* **140** (4), 1097 (1989).
13. L. Beck, Jr. and P. A. D'Amore, Vascular development: cellular and molecular regulation, *Faseb J* **11** (5), 365 (1997).
14. N. Takakura, T. Watanabe, S. Suenobu, Y. Yamada, T. Noda, Y. Ito, M. Satake, and T. Suda, A role for hematopoietic stem cells in promoting angiogenesis, *Cell* **102** (2), 199 (2000).
15. J. R. Crosby, W. E. Kaminski, G. Schatteman, P. J. Martin, E. W. Raines, R. A. Seifert, and D. F. Bowen-Pope, Endothelial cells of hematopoietic origin make a significant contribution to adult blood vessel formation, *Circ Res* **87** (9), 728 (2000).
16. T. Murohara, H. Ikeda, J. Duan, S. Shintani, Ki Sasaki, H. Eguchi, I. Onitsuka, K. Matsui, and T. Imaizumi, Transplanted cord blood-derived endothelial precursor cells augment postnatal neovascularization, *J Clin Invest* **105** (11), 1527 (2000).
17. C. Müller-Sieburg, ed., Hematopoietic stem cells: animal models and human transplantation, in *Current Topics in Microbiology and Immunology* (Springer-Verlag, New York, 1992), Vol. 177.
18. D. E. Harrison, C. T. Jordan, R. K. Zhong, and C. M. Astle, Primitive hemopoietic stem cells: direct assay of most productive populations by competitive repopulation with simple binomial, correlation and covariance calculations, *Exp Hematol* **21** (2), 206 (1993).
19. M. A. Goodell, K. A. Jackson, S. M. Majka, T. Mi, H. Wang, J. Pocius, C. J. Hartley, M. W. Majesky, M. L. Entman, L. H. Michael, and K. K. Hirschi, Stem cell plasticity in muscle and bone marrow, *Ann N Y Acad Sci* **938**, 208 (2001).

20. D. S. Krause, N. D. Theise, M. I. Collector, O. Henegariu, S. Hwang, R. Gardner, S. Neutzel, and S. J. Sharkis, Multi-organ, multi-lineage engraftment by a single bone marrow-derived stem cell, *Cell* **105** (3), 369 (2001).
21. B. E. Petersen, W. C. Bowen, K. D. Patrene, W. M. Mars, A. K. Sullivan, N. Murase, S. S. Boggs, J. S. Greenberger, and J. P. Goff, Bone marrow as a potential source of hepatic oval cells, *Science* **284** (5417), 1168 (1999).
22. E. Lagasse, H. Connors, M. Al-Dhalimy, M. Reitsma, M. Dohse, L. Osborne, X. Wang, M. Finegold, I. L. Weissman, and M. Grompe, Purified hematopoietic stem cells can differentiate into hepatocytes in vivo, *Nat Med* **6** (11), 1229 (2000).
23. D. Orlic, J. Kajstura, S. Chimenti, I. Jakoniuk, S. M. Anderson, B. Li, J. Pickel, R. McKay, B. Nadal-Ginard, D. M. Bodine, A. Leri, and P. Anversa, Bone marrow cells regenerate infarcted myocardium, *Nature* **410** (6829), 701 (2001).
24. M. B. Grant, W. S. May, S. Caballero, G. A. Brown, S. M. Guthrie, R. N. Mames, B. J. Byrne, T. Vaught, P. E. Spoerri, A. B. Peck, and E. W. Scott, Adult hematopoietic stem cells provide functional hemangioblast activity during retinal neovascularization, *Nat Med* **8** (6), 607 (2002).
25. C. Kalka, H. Tehrani, B. Laudenberg, P. R. Vale, J. M. Isner, T. Asahara, and J. F. Symes, VEGF gene transfer mobilizes endothelial progenitor cells in patients with inoperable coronary disease, *Ann Thorac Surg* **70** (3), 829 (2000).
26. J. Llevadot, S. Murasawa, Y. Kureishi, S. Uchida, H. Masuda, A. Kawamoto, K. Walsh, J. M. Isner, and T. Asahara, HMG-CoA reductase inhibitor mobilizes bone marrow--derived endothelial progenitor cells, *J Clin Invest* **108** (3), 399 (2001).
27. S. J. Sharkis, S. Neutzel, and M. I. Collector, Phenotype and function of hematopoietic stem cells, *Ann N Y Acad Sci* **938**, 191 (2001).
28. O. N. Koc, S. L. Gerson, B. W. Cooper, S. M. Dyhouse, S. E. Haynesworth, A. I. Caplan, and H. M. Lazarus, Rapid hematopoietic recovery after coinfusion of autologous-blood stem cells and culture-expanded marrow mesenchymal stem cells in advanced breast cancer patients receiving high-dose chemotherapy, *J Clin Oncol* **18** (2), 307 (2000).
29. J. D. Mosca, J. K. Hendricks, D. Buyaner, J. Davis-Sproul, L. C. Chuang, M. K. Majumdar, R. Chopra, F. Barry, M. Murphy, M. A. Thiede, U. Junker, R. J. Rigg, S. P. Forestell, E. Bohnlein, R. Storb, and B. M. Sandmaier, Mesenchymal stem cells as vehicles for gene delivery, *Clin Orthop* (379 Suppl), S71 (2000).
30. D. Cilloni, C. Carlo-Stella, F. Falzetti, G. Sammarelli, E. Regazzi, S. Colla, V. Rizzoli, F. Aversa, M. F. Martelli, and A. Tabilio, Limited engraftment capacity of bone marrow-derived mesenchymal cells following T-cell-depleted hematopoietic stem cell transplantation, *Blood* **96** (10), 3637 (2000).
31. S. M. Devine, A. M. Bartholomew, N. Mahmud, M. Nelson, S. Patil, W. Hardy, C. Sturgeon, T. Hewett, T. Chung, W. Stock, D. Sher, S. Weissman, K. Ferrer, J. Mosca, R. Deans, A. Moseley, and R. Hoffman, Mesenchymal stem cells are capable of homing to the bone marrow of non- human primates following systemic infusion, *Exp Hematol* **29** (2), 244 (2001).
32. O. N. Koc, C. Peters, P. Aubourg, S. Raghavan, S. Dyhouse, R. DeGasperi, E. H. Kolodny, Y. B. Yoseph, S. L. Gerson, H. M. Lazarus, A. I. Caplan, P. A. Watkins, and W. Krivit, Bone marrow-derived mesenchymal stem cells remain host-derived despite successful hematopoietic engraftment after allogeneic transplantation in patients with lysosomal and peroxisomal storage diseases, *Exp Hematol* **27** (11), 1675 (1999).

IN VITRO TRANSFORMATION OF MONOCYTES AND DENDRITIC CELLS INTO ENDOTHELIAL LIKE CELLS

Klaus Havemann, Beatriz F. Pujol, and Jürgen Adamkiewicz[*]

1. SUMMARY

Our *in vitro* data indicate that peripheral blood monocytes or monocyte-derived immature dendritic cells under appropriate culture conditions transdifferentiate into endothelial-like cells (ELC), which are characterized by the expression of endothelial markers and the formation of tube-like structures. Dependent on the culture conditions a mixed macrophage/endothelial or an endothelial phenotype could be induced. A similar pattern of development could be seen in $CD14^+$ monocyte-derived ELC and ELC grown from $CD34^+$ precursor cells or from dendritic cells generated from $CD34^+$ cells. These *in vitro* data suggest that monocytes are precursors of different subgroups of endothelial cells and that the formation of endothelial cells from $CD34^+$ progenitor cells follows a similar pathway possibly via the monocyte and/or the immature dendritic cell.

2. TRANSDIFFERENTIATION POTENTIAL OF MONOCYTES

The macrophage is thought to be the major terminally differentiated cell type of the mononuclear phagocyte system. Macrophages and neutrophils share a common bone marrow derived progenitor cell, the CFU-GM, which becomes committed to one or the other differentiation pathway at an early stage. Monocytes/macrophages have intimate contact with the vascular system (Leek et al., 1997). Tissue macrophages originate from blood monocytes that migrate via chemotactic signals through the endothelial cell layer. This is achieved by adherence to the endothelium utilizing surface glycoproteins such as CD11a and ICAM-1. In addition macrophages produce a broad spectrum of angiogenesis modulating factors including cytokines and ECM degrading enzymes, which induce angiogenesis and promote endothelial cell migration (Leek et al., 1997).

In the 1920s Ludwig Aschoff postulated a common origin of macrophages and endothelial cells which he united in the so-called reticulo-endothelial system (Aschoff, 1924). However, until recently analyses of a direct relationship between the monocyte/macrophage and the endothelial system had not been reactivated. The concept of stem cell biology during the last decades was that precursor cells proliferate and differentiate in an irreversible process to

---

[*] Institute of Molecular Biology and Tumor Research, Philipps University, Marburg, Germany

Novel Angiogenic Mechanisms: Role of Circulating Progenitor Endothelial Cells.
Edited by Nicanor I. Moldovan, Kluwer Academic/Plenum Publishers, 2003.

terminally differentiated cells. However, recent experiments have demonstrated the surprising capacity of more mature cells to dedifferentiate. Thus, this rather inflexible concept has been replaced by the present view: cells including more differentiated ones have a recruitable but decreasing propensity to act as stem cells as they differentiate (Blau et al., 2001). The traditional concept of the terminally differentiated cell is further weakened by experiments demonstrating that the differentiated state in adult mammalian cells is not fixed and irreversible, but instead is regulated by a dynamic active process that requires continuous regulation. This process of transdifferentiation is defined as a phenotypic modulation, in general without any need for cell division. There are many surprising examples of transdifferentiation, as for example the transformation of exocrine pancreas duct cells into insulin secreting β-cells (Bouwens et al., 1998). Also, the blood monocyte under the influence of various cytokines is known to transdifferentiate *in vitro* and *in vivo* into morphologically and functionally different cells (Figure 1). Depending on the composition of growth and differentiation factors in the surrounding milieu the monocyte transforms into such different cells as macrophages, dendritic cells, osteoclasts and possibly also osteoblasts (Zhou et al., 1996; Nicholson et al., 2000; Heinemann et al., 2000).

3. TRANSDIFFERENTIATION OF MONOCYTES AND DENDRITIC CELLS INTO ENDOTHELIAL-LIKE CELLS

Here we present *in vitro* data on transdifferentiation of human $CD14^+$ monocytes and monocyte-derived dendritic cells into endothelial-like cells (ELC), suggesting a direct role of monocytes in angiogenesis (Pujol et al., 2000a; Pujol et al., 2001). This hypothesis is supported by results of other groups (Moldovan et al., 2000; Kalka et al., 2000; Schmeisser et al., 2001; Harraz et al., 2001), who have described either a similar transformational process *in vitro* or even a participation of blood monocytes in experimental neoangiogenesis *in vivo*.

Since the publication of Asahara et al. (1996) on the generation of endothelial cell precursors from enriched $CD34^+$ cells, many groups confirmed that $CD34^+$ stem cells from bone marrow or peripheral blood are able to form endothelial cells *in vitro* and *in vivo*. Asahara described a typical oval or spindle shape appearance of these adherent cells.

Our group also described these typical cells with endothelial cell markers, when we cultured total mononuclear cells from peripheral blood. We then separated the different cell populations of mononuclear cells, and to our surprise, could show that only peripheral monocytes were able to form these endothelial like cells (Pujol et al., 2000a). We therefore concentrated our attempts on highly purified $CD14^+$ human blood monocytes, which we obtained by magnetic cell separation. FACS analysis of this starting population showed >95% $CD14^+$ and $CD45^+$ cells. These were cultured with growth factors and cytokines to obtain either macrophages, dendritic cells, or endothelial like cells. Macrophages were generated with M-CSF, dendritic cells with GM-CSF and IL-4, and endothelial like cells with endothelial growth medium containing VEGF, bFGF, IGF-1, hydrocortisone and FCS, the latter cells were kept on Fibronectin coated surfaces. Macrophages and dendritic cells exhibited their typical morphology, whereas endothelial like cells showed adherent oval or spindle shaped cells.

Immunohistochemical staining of these different cell populations was compared with HUVEC and HMVEC as shown in Table 1. Macrophages exhibited the typical markers CD14, CD68, and non-specific esterase as well as markers of antigen presenting cells, but did not express specific endothelial markers such as von Willebrand factor or VE-cadherin. Dendritic cells strongly expressed CD1a, CD83, markers of antigen presenting cells and, to some extent, also of macrophage markers. To our surprise, however, they also showed a weak staining for vWF and VE-cadherin. Endothelial like cells, on the other hand, expressed a number of endothelial markers including vWF and VE-cadherin, macrophage markers and markers of antigen presenting cells, whereas they did not stain for dendritic cell markers. This mixed macrophage/endothelial cell phenotype of endothelial like cells was confirmed by PCR analysis, where the cells expressed CD14, vWF, CD36, and Flt-1 mRNA, but only very weakly KDR mRNA. Ultrastructural analyses revealed secretory granules with a wide size range. At higher magnification some of the compact inclusions exhibited highly ordered lamellar structures resembling Weibel-Palade bodies, the storage granules of vWF. In long term culture the cells formed network-like structures.

Apart from the generation of hybrid cells with both macrophage and endothelial cell markers, these results also suggest the existence of some relationship between endothelial like cells and dendritic cells, especially in their immature form.

We therefore generated immature dendritic cells with GM-CSF and IL-4 (Table 2), cells which strongly expressed CD1a but not CD83, and which showed a moderate staining for the endothelial specific markers vWF and VE-cadherin. These cells were then cultured with the same cytokines but with addition of TNFα. As expected, the cells now expressed CD83, the marker of mature dendritic cells, and markedly reduced their CD1a expression. Again, these cells showed a moderate expression of the endothelial cell markers.

On the other hand, when immature dendritic cells were cultured with endothelial cell growth medium containing angiogenic factors on Fibronectin coated surfaces, again a mixed macrophage/endothelial phenotype of strongly adherent cells without dendritic cell markers was obtained (Table 2)

We then speculated that IL-4, an anti-inflammatory cytokine with inhibitory effects on macrophage function that induces endothelial cell formation, might be essential for endothelial cell growth. After testing different cytokines, we combined IL-4 with oncostatin M, an early response protein of the IL-6 family, which has pleiotrophic effects on different cell systems including the differentiation of endothelial cells.

When CD14$^+$ cells were grown, either from the beginning or after pre-culture with GM-CSF and IL-4, in endothelial growth medium supplemented with Il-4 and oncostatin M (Table 2, Figure 2), a homogeneous population of oval cells appeared with no signs of dendritic cell or macrophage differentiation. In addition, these cells were negative for non-specific esterase. They were characterized by the disappearance of CD14, CD1a and CD83, and by the expression of Ac-LDL receptor, vWF, KDR and Flt-4 as shown by immunohistochemistry and PCR analysis. VE-cadherin expression clearly increased and for the first time some CD34 positive cells could be demonstrated. The oval slightly adherent cells with some small cytoplasmic extensions built numerous clusters, cobblestones and in prolonged cultures tube-like structures on a plasma gel.

Although these cells exhibited a significantly reduced capacity to prime T-cells when compared to mature dendritic cells, a distinct change of expression of HLA-DR and CD86 could not be shown.

These results suggest a close relationship between immature dendritic cells and the endothelial like cells described here. In contrast to the aforementioned endothelial like cells characterized by a mixed macrophage/endothelial phenotype, these cells resemble much more endothelial cells. The expression of the thrombospondin receptor CD36 may indicate their relationship to the microvascular phenotype.

4. DIFFERENTIATION OF CD34$^+$ PROGENITOR CELLS INTO ENDOTHELIAL-LIKE CELLS

To what extent are these *in vitro* results in accordance with the known ability of CD34[+] progenitor cells to form endothelial cells? Is the blood monocyte during the differentiation of CD34[+] progenitor cells perhaps an interim cell for the development of either macrophages, dendritic cells or endothelial cells?

To address this question, we cultured human CD34[+] progenitor cells obtained by magnetic separation from peripheral blood of G-CSF mobilised donors (Pujol et al., 2000b). Again, the cells were cultured with GM-CSF and IL-4 to generate dendritic cells, or in the presence of angiogenic growth factors to obtain endothelial like cells. The starting populations were of high purity expressing CD34, CD38, CD45, HLA-DR, but not CD14. When we cultured the cells in endothelial cell growth medium on Fibronectin coated slides (Table 3) we again obtained, as shown before, a mixed macrophage/endothelial phenotype with strongly adherent oval and large oval cells with a moderate expression of vWF and VE-cadherin, but no expression of dendritic cell markers.

Immature dendritic cells clearly positive for CD1a but without expression of CD83 were raised with GM-CSF/IL-4. Similar to the results obtained with blood monocytes, these cells also weakly expressed vWF and VE-cadherin. Upon addition of TNFα the maturation marker CD83 could be demonstrated. When the immature dendritic cells were cultured with endothelial cell growth medium containing angiogenic growth factors (Table 4), again strongly adherent oval and large oval cells could be generated which showed the known mixed macrophage/endothelial phenotype.

However, when CD34[+] progenitor cells were cultured in the presence of angiogenic growth factors together with GM-CSF/IL-4 or IL-4/Oncostatin M, slightly adherent oval cells with cluster and network formation were raised which showed a high expression of the endothelial markers vWF and VE-cadherin (Table 4). When cultured with IL-4/oncostatin M, the cells lost their CD36 expression.

The only differences between cultures starting from CD34[+] cells and those starting from blood monocytes were the lower expression of HLA-DR and CD86, and a moderate cell proliferation as indicated by an increase in cell density.

5. IN VIVO CORRELATES OF ENDOTHELIAL-LIKE CELLS GROWN IN VITRO

Which are the possible *in vivo* correlates of these different endothelial like cells generated *in vitro*? Many publications show that macrovascular endothelial cells strongly express VEGF-receptor 1/KDR, vWF, and VE-cadherin (Mutin et al., 1997). On the other hand, microvascular endothelial cells are characterized by the thrombospondin receptor CD36 and the expression of CD80, CD86, and HLA-DR, which are markers of antigen presenting cells (Swerlick et al., 1992; Mc Douall et al., 1996). Sinus lining cells probably have a mixed macrophage/endothelial phenotype (Krenacs et al., 1995; Uccini et al., 1997), whereas the related endothelial cells of the lymphatic system typically exhibit Flt-4, the VEGF-receptor 3 (Paavonen et al., 2000). Our data suggest that depending on culture conditions predominantly endothelial like cells either of the sinus lining or the microvascular phenotype have been grown *in vitro*.

The paradigm that postnatal angiogenesis is exclusively caused by outgrowth of endothelial cells from preformed vessels has to be modified according to the recent findings. In addition to this mechanism, circulating CD34[+] stem cells and probably also peripheral monocytes and immature dendritic cells may participate in postnatal angiogenesis. Furthermore, our *in vitro* data suggest that the formation of endothelial cells from CD34[+] precursor cells may follow a similar pathway via monocytes or monocyte precursors or via immature dendritic cells.

6. REFERENCES

Asahara, T., Murohara, T., Sullivan, A., Silver, M., van der Zee, R., Li, T., Witzenbichler, B., Schatteman, G., and Isner, J. M., 1997, Isolation of putative progenitor endothelial cells for angiogenesis, *Science* **275**: 964.

Aschoff, L., 1924, Das reticuloendotheliale System, *Erg. Inn. Med. Kinderheilk.* **26**:1.

Blau, H. M., Brazelton, T. R., and Weimann, J. M., 2001, The evolving concept of a stem cell: entity or function, *Cell* **105**: 829.

Bouwens, L., 1998, Transdifferentiation versus stem cell hypothesis for the regeneration of islet beta-cells in the pancreas, *Microsc Res Tech* **43**: 332.

Harraz, M., Jiao, C., Hanlon, H. D., Hartley, R. S., and Schatteman, G. C., 2001, CD34(-) blood derived human endothelial cell progenitors, *Stem Cells* **19**: 304.

Heinemann, D. E., Siggelkow, H., Ponce, L. M., Viereck, Y., Wiese K. G., and Peters J. H., 2000, Alkaline phosphatase expression during monocyte differentiation. Overlapping markers as a link between monocytic cells, dendritic cells, osteoclasts and osteoblasts, *Immunobiology* **202**: 68.

Kalka, C., Masuda, H., Takahashi, T., Kalka-Moll, W. M., Silver, M., Kearney, M., Li, T., Isner, J. M., and Asahara, T., 2000, Transplantation of *ex vivo* expanded endothelial progenitor cells for therapeutic neovascularisation, *Proc Nat A Sci USA* **97**: 3422.

Krenacs, T., and Rosendaal, M., 1995, Immunohistochemical detection of gap junctions in human lymphoid tissue: connexin 43 in follicular dendritic and lymphoendothelial cells, *J Histochem Cytochem* **43**: 1125.

Leek, R. D., Lewis, C. E., and Harris, A. L., 1997, The role of macrophages in tumor angiogenesis, in: *Tumor Angiogenesis*, R. Bicknell, C. E. Lewis, and N. Ferrara, eds, Oxford University Press, Oxford, pp. 81-91.

McDouall, R. M., Yacoub, M., and Rose, M. L., 1996, Isolation, culture and characterisation of MHC class II-positive microvascular endothelial cells from the human heart, *Microvasc Res* **51**: 137.

Moldovan, N. J., Goldschmidt-Clermont, P. J., Parker-Thornburg, J., Shapiro, S. D., and Kolattukudy, P. E., 2000, Contribution of monocytes/macrophages to compensatory neovascularisation. The drilling of metalloelastase-positive tunnels in ischemic myocardium, *Circ Res* **87**:378.

Mutin, M., Dignat-George, F., and Sampol, J., 1997, Immunologic phenotype of cultured endothelial cells: quantitative analysis of cell surface molecules, *Tissue Antigens* **50**: 449.

Nicholson, G. C., Malakellis, M., Collier, F. M., Cameron, P. K., Holloway, W. R., Gough, T. J., Gregorio-King, C., Kirkland, M. A., and Meyers, D. E., 2000, Induction of osteoclasts from CD14-positive human peripheral blood mononuclear cells by receptor activator of nuclear factor kappa B ligand (RANKL), *Clin Sci* **99**: 133.

Paavonen, K., Puolakkasinen, P., Jussila, L., Jahkola, T., and Alitalo, K., 2000, Vascular endothelial cell growth factor receptor-3 in lymphangiogenesis and wound healing, *Am J Pathol* **156**: 1499.

Pujol, B. F., Lucibello, F. C., Gehling, U. M., Lindemann, K., Weidner, N., Zuzarte, M. L., Adamkiewicz, J., Elsässer, H. P., Müller, R., and Havemann, K., 2000a, Endothelial-like cells derived from CD14 positive monocytes, *Differentiation* **65**: 287.

Pujol, B. F., Lucibello, F. C., Zuzarte, M. L., Lütjens, P., Müller, R., and Havemann, K., 2001, Dendritic cells derived from peripheral monocytes express endothelial markers and in the presence of angiogenic growth factors differentiate into endothelial-like cells, *Eur J Cell Biol* **80**: 99.

Pujol, B. F., Lucibello, F. C., Zuzarte, M. L., Müller, R., and Havemann, K., 2000b, Dendritic cells (DC) generated from hematopoietic progenitor cells express endothelial cell markers and can be converted into endothelial like cells (ELC) in the presence of angiogenic growth factors, *Proc Am A Canc R* **41**: 116.

Schmeisser, A., Garlichs, C. D., Zhang, H., Eskafi, S., Graffy, C., Ludwig, J., Strasser, R. H., and Daniel, W. G., 2001, Monocytes coexpress endothelial and macrophagocytic lineage markers and form cord-like structures in matrigel under angiogenic conditions, *Cardiovasc Res* **49**: 671.

Swerlick, R. A., Lee, K. H., Wick, T.M., and Lawley, T. J., 1992, Human dermal microvascular endothelial but not human umbilical vein endothelial cells express CD36 in vivo and in vitro, *J Immunol* **148**: 78.

Uccini, S., Sirianni, M. C., Vincenzi, L., Topino, S., Stoppacciaro, A., Lesnoni La Parola, I., Capuano, M., Masini, C., Cerimele, D., Cella, M., Lanzavecchia, A., Allavena, P., Mantovani, A., Baroni, C. D., and Ruco, L. P., 1997, Kaposi`s sarcoma cells express the macrophage-associated antigen mannose receptor and develop in peripheral blood cultures of Kaposi`s sarcoma patients, *Am J Pathol* **150**: 929.

Zhou, L. J., and Tedder, T. F., 1996, CD14+ blood monocytes can differentiate into functionally mature CD83+ dendritic cells, *Proc Natl Acad Sci USA* **93**: 2588.

                                                  K. HAVEMANN *ET AL.*

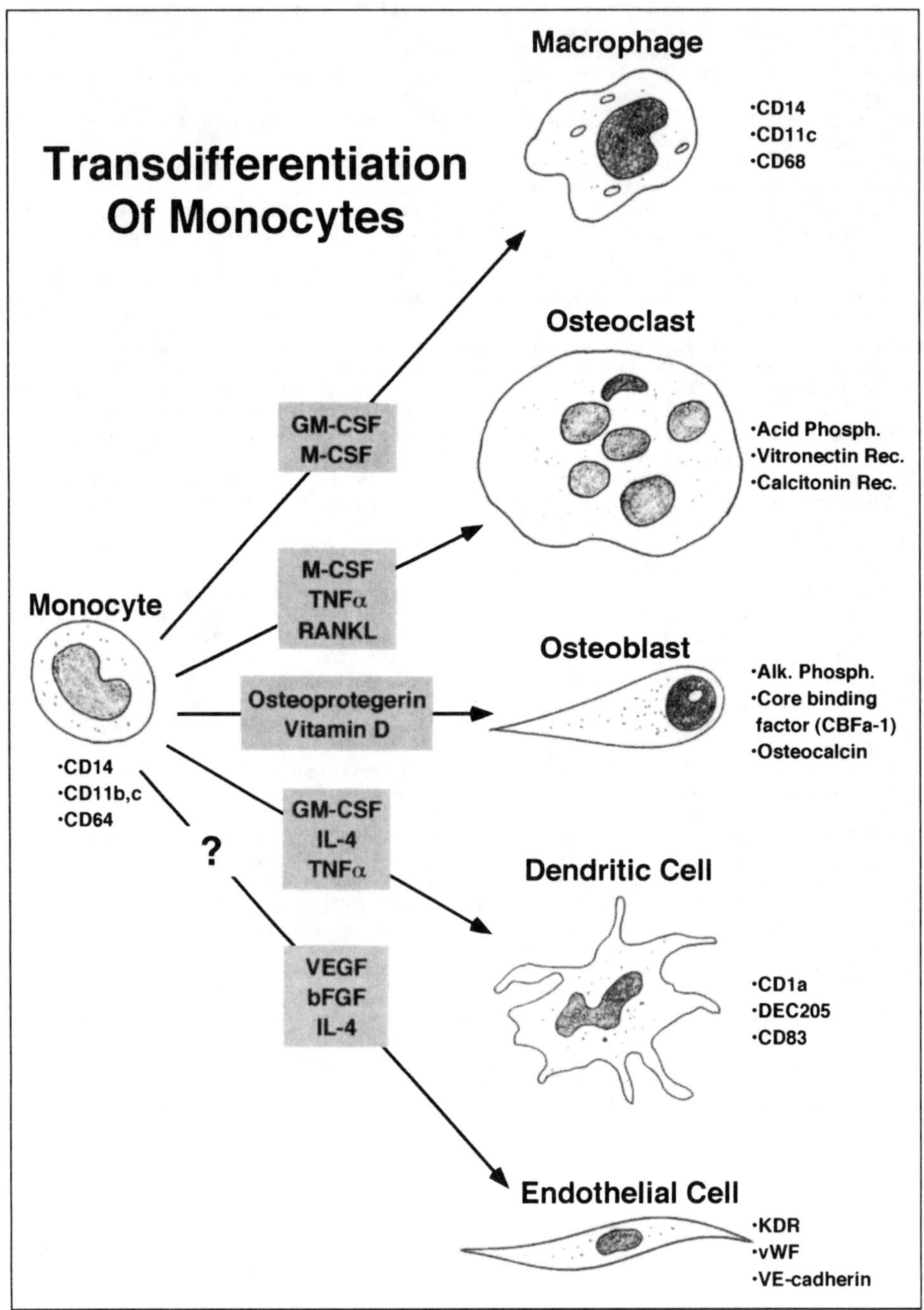

Figure 1. Transdifferentiation pathways of monocytes.

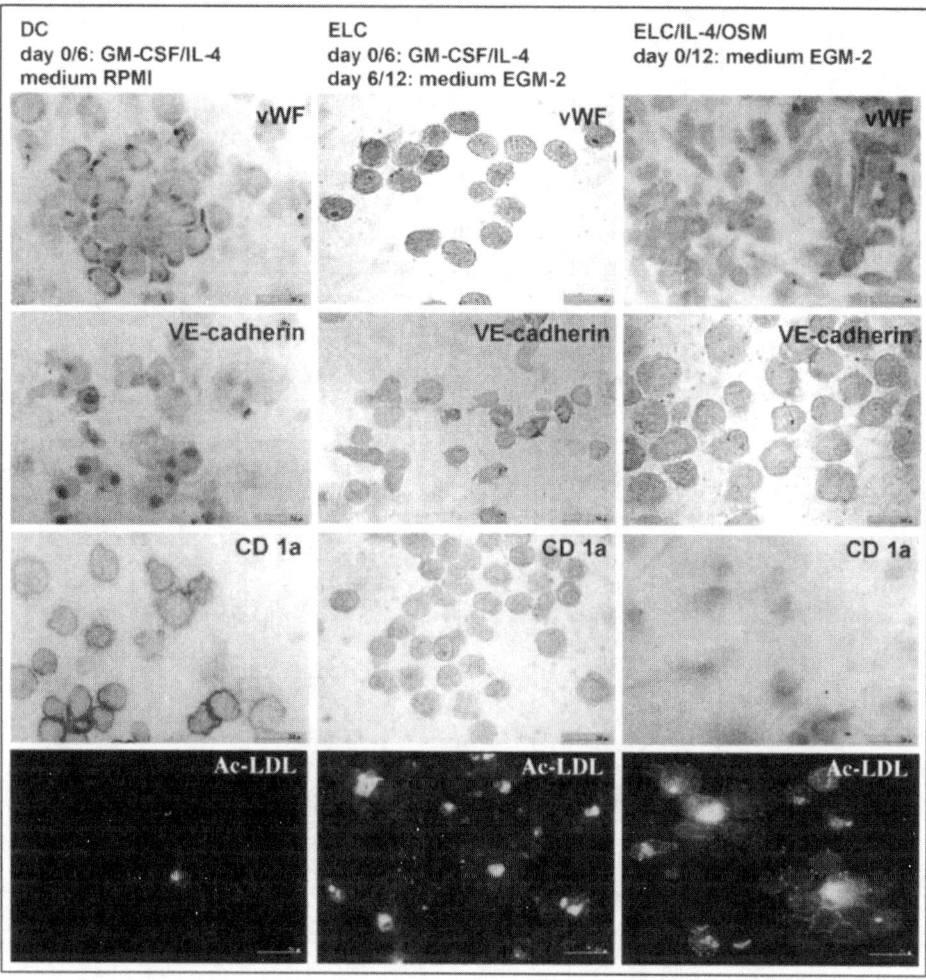

Figure 2. Immunohistochemical characterisation of CD14$^+$ cells grown in endothelial growth medium supplemented with IL-4 and oncostatin M. For a color representation of this figure, see color insert at the end of book.

Table 1. Results of immunocytochemistry (APAAP)

Markers (M)		HUVEC	HMVEC	Macrophages M-CSF d12	Dendritic cells GM-CSF/IL-4 d12	Endothel. like cells EGM II/VEGF d12
Endothel.-M.	CD31	+	++	+++	++	++
	CD34	++[a]	+[a]	Ø	Ø	Ø*
	CD36	Ø	+/++	+[a,b]	+[a]	+/++[b]
	CD54	++	+/++	+[a]	n.d.	+/++[b]
	CD105	++	++	++	n.d.	++
	VE-Cadherin	++	++	Ø*	+[a,b]	+[b]
	vWF	++	+/++[a]	Ø*	+[a]	+/++[b]
Macroph. M.	CD14	Ø	Ø	++[b]	Ø*	+[a]
	CD68	++	++	+++	++	++/+++
	Esterase	Ø	Ø	++	+[a]	++
DC-M	CD1a	Ø	Ø	Ø*	++[b]	Ø*
	CD83	Ø	Ø	Ø	+/++[a]	Ø
APC-M	CD86	Ø	+	++	++	++
	HLA-DR	Ø	+	++[b]	++/+++	++

Ø negative, + moderate stain, ++ strong stain, +++ very strong stain   * < 5%, [a] 10-30%, [b] 30-50%, no index 50-100% positive, n.d. not done. DC dendritic cells, APC antigen presenting cells

Table 2. Culture of CD14[+] cells (day 6, day 7-12). Results of immunocytochemistry

DC, immature (RPMI, GM-CSF,IL-4) ⇒ **DC, mature (RPMI, GM-CSF, IL-4, TNFα)**

	Morph.	CD1a	CD83	vWF	CD144	CD86	HLA-DR	CD36	CD34
Total cells	OC,DC	+/++[a,b]	+/++[a,b]	+[b]	+[a,b]	++/++	++/+++	+[a,b]	∅

⇒ **ELC (EGM, VEGF, Fibronectin)**

	Morph.	CD1a	CD83	vWF	CD144	CD86	HLA-DR	CD36	CD34
Total cells	OC,LOC	∅[*]	∅[*]	+/++[b]	+[a]	++	+++	+/++[a]	∅

⇒ **ELC (EGM, VEGF, IL-4, OSM, Fibronectin)**

	Morph.	CD1a	CD83	vWF	CD144	CD86	HLA-DR	CD36	CD34
Adh.cells	OC, Clust.	∅	∅[*]	+[b]	+/++[a,b]	++/+++	+++	+/++[a]	∅
Sup.cells	OC, Clust.	∅	∅	+[a]	++[b]	n.d.	n.d.	n.d.	n.d.

ELC (EGM,VEGF, IL-4, OSM, Fibronectin) ⇒ **ELC (EGM, VEGF, IL-4, OSM, Fibronectin)**

	Morph.	CD1a	CD83	vWF	CD144	CD86	HLA-DR	CD36	CD34
Adh.cells	OC, Clust Network	∅	∅[*]	+[b]	++[b]	++	++[b]	+[b]	+[a]
Sup.cells	OC,Clust	∅	∅	+/++[a]	++[b]	++	+[b]	n.d.	n.d.

Day 0-6   Day 7-12

EGM: endothelial cell growth medium II (VEGF, bFGF, IGF-1, 10% FCS,5% horse serum) RPMI:RPMI+10%FCS   OSM: Oncostatin M. DC: dendritic cells, ELC: endothelial like cells, OC: oval cells, LOC: large OC, Clust: cluster. ∅ negative, + moderate stain, ++ strong stain, +++ very strong stain, [*] <5%,. [a] 10-30%, [b] 30-50%, no index 50-100% positive.

Table 3. Culture of CD34[+] cells (day 6, day 7-12).   Results of immunocytochemistry

Day 0-6

VEGF (EGM-2, 10% FCS, Fibronectin

Morph.	CD1a	CD83	vWF	CD144	CD86	HLA-DR	CD36
SC, OC	Ø*	Ø	+[a]	+[b]	+/++[b]	++	++[b]

GM-CSF/IL-4 (RPMI, 10% FCS)

Morph.	CD1a	CD83	vWF	CD144	CD86	HLA-DR	CD36
OC	++[a]	Ø*	+[a,b]	+[b]	+/++[a,b]	+/++[b]	Ø
CL+							

⇒

Day 7-12

VEGF (EGM-2, 10% FCS, Fibronectin)

Morph.	CD1a	CD83	vWF	CD144	CD86	HLA-DR	CD36
OC, SC, LOC	Ø*	Ø	+/++[a,b]	+[a,b]	++	++	++[b]
MLOC							

GM-CSF/IL-4/TNFα (RPMI, 10%FCS)

Morph.	CD1a	CD83	vWF	CD144	CD86	HLA-DR	CD36
OC, DC	++[a,b]	+/++[a,b]	+[a,b]	+[a]	++	++/+++	Ø*
CL++							

VEGF (EGM-2, 10% FCS, Fibronectin)

Morph.	CD1a	CD83	vWF	CD144	CD86	HLA-DR	CD36
OC, SC, LOC	Ø*	Ø	+[a]	+[a,b]	++	++	+/++[b]
MLOL							

AC: adherent cells, SC: supernatant cells, OC: oval cells, LOC: large oval cells, ML0C: multinucleated LOC, CL: cluster.   Ø negative, + moderate stain, ++ strong stain, +++ very strong stain, * < 5%, [a] 10-30%, [b] 30-50%, no index 50-100% positive

Table 4. Culture of CD34[+] cells (day 7-10).   Results of immunocytochemistry

DC GM-CSF/Il-4 (RPMI, 10% FCS)

	CD1a	CD83	vWF	CD144	CD86	HLA-DR	CD36
SC	++[a]	Ø[*]	+[a,b]	+[b]	+/++[a,b]	+/++[b]	Ø[*]

Comment: Immature DC without expression of CD83 and CD36 and weak expression of vWF/CD144

ELC VEGF/GM-CSF/IL-4 (EGM-2, 10% FCS, Fibronectin)

	CD1a	CD83	vWF	CD144	CD86	HLA-DR	CD36
AC	Ø[*]	Ø	Ø-+[a]	+[a]	++	+++	++
SC	Ø[*]	Ø	++	+/++	++[b]	++	+/++[b]

Comment: 1. Strongly adherent macrophages (LOC, MLOC, CD36+)
            2. Loosly adherent CD36+ ELC (OC) with marked proliferation (increase of cell density and cluster formation), moderate expression of vWF/CD144

ELC VEGF/IL-4/Oncostatin M (EGM-2, 10% FCS, Fibronectin)

	CD1a	CD83	vWF	CD144	CD86	HLA-DR	CD36
AC	Ø[*]	Ø	Ø	+[a]	++[b]	++[b]	Ø[*]
SC	Ø[*]	Ø	++	++	+/++[a]	++[b]	Ø

Comment: Loosely adherent ELC with no CD36 and decreased HLA-DR/CD86 expression, highest expression of vWF/CD144, moderate proliferation.

AC: adherent cells, SC: supernatant cells.   Ø negative, + moderate stain, ++ strong stain, +++ very strong stain, * < 5%, [a] 10-30%, [b] 30-50%, no index 50-100% positive.

PHENOTYPIC OVERLAP BETWEEN MONOCYTES AND VASCULAR ENDOTHELIAL CELLS

Alexander Schmeisser, Christiane Graffy, Werner G. Daniel, and Ruth H. Strasser, MD*

1. SUMMARY

During embryonic development, endothelial cells (ECs) develop organ specific properties. ECs express specific markers, which are helpful in identifying these cells in vivo and in culture. Interestingly, most of the supposed specific endothelial markers are present on both ECs and hematopoietic precursors or mature blood cells, which correspond to the idea of a common embryonic precursor. Monocytes/makrophages and monocyte-derived dendritic cells, as more differentiated hematopoietic cell populations, show a wide phenotypic overlap with particularly hepatic sinusoidal, and microvascular endothelial cells within inflamed tissue, such as neovascularizised complicated atherosclerotic plaques. Furthermore, under local angiogenic growth conditions monocytes or monocyte precursors or immature dendritic cells may differentiate into endothelial like cells. First evidence suggests an endothelium-independent revascularization potential carried by monocyte-derived macrophages. These macrophages have been shown to form tunnel-like structures in ischemic regions. Future studies have to address the question, whether monocyte-/dendritic cell-derived endothelial like cells can develop a similar functional behaviour in vasoregulation, coagulation and fibrinolysis, as described for vascular endothelial cells, and thus may contribute to neoangiogenesis by a direct vessel-forming role.

2. INTRODUCTION

During embryonic development, endothelial cells develop organ specific properties. The acquisition and maintenance of specialized properties by endothelial cells is important in the functional homeostasis of the different organs. ECs express specific

---

* Department of Cardiology, Medical Clinic II, University of Technology Dresden, Fetscherstr. 76, D-01307 Dresden, Christiane Graffy and Werner G. Daniel Medical Clinic II Friedrich Alexander University, Erlangen-Nuernberg, Oestliche Stadtmauerstr. 29, D-91054 Erlangen, Germany

Novel Angiogenic Mechanisms: Role of Circulating Progenitor Endothelial Cells.
Edited by Nicanor I. Moldovan, Kluwer Academic/Plenum Publishers, 2003.

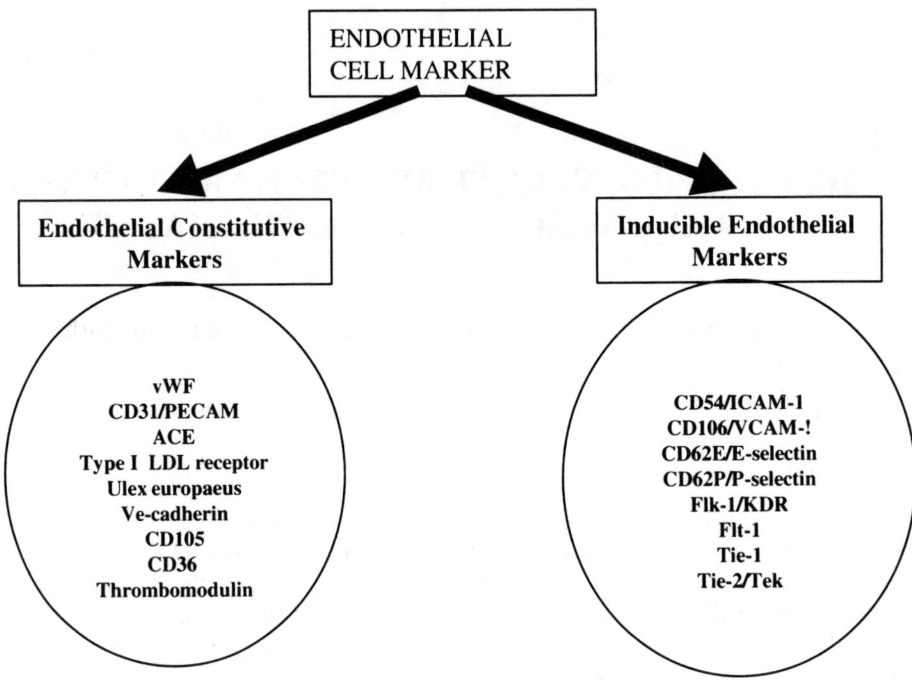

Figure 1. Examples for constitutive and inducible endothelial cell marker

markers which are helpful in identifying these cells in vivo and in culture (eg. von Willebrand factor, VE-cadherin, Ulex europaeus, CD105). Some of the EC markers are constitutive and present in essentially all types of endothelium. Other molecules are expressed only after activation by inflammatory cytokines or growth factors. (Figure 1.) Some markers are rather specific for EC of different origins, such as from the brain and blood brain barrier (BBB) or bone marrow or the lymphatic system.[1,2] This last category is relatively scarce, because EC isolation from the microvasculature of certain vascular regions is still technically difficult, and once in culture, they tend to lose their specialized properties (references in 1). Only in the past few years the technology has become available which permits the in situ study of ECs. New techniques are under development such as the injection of phage-display peptide libraries, which detect specific surface molecules in the peripheral endothelium in vivo.[1]

Interestingly, most of the supposed specific endothelial markers are present on both ECs and hematopoietic precursors or mature blood cells, which correspond to the idea of a common embryonic precursor.[3-5] Recently, several lines of evidence suggest the existence of circulating endothelial precursor cells in adult organisms.[6-9] In summary these data indicate, that only a very small subset of circulating hematopoietic (stem?) cells expressing the surface markers AC133 and/or AC133/Flk-1/CD34, have the capacity to differentiate into endothelial cells. This indicates that these cells represent angioblast-like circulating endothelial progenitor cells. They coexpress common endothelial and hematopoietic antigens. Among these phenotypic overlap, AC133 is suggested as the only marker to differentiate between the circulating endothelial progenitor cells and mature endothelial cells. [10-17] (Table 1.)

Asahara et al.[6, 18] described also the in vitro formation of an endothelial progenitor cell population (EPC). But they were formed by on plastic adherent mononuclear (monocytes?) cells of human peripheral blood enriched with ~ 16% CD34-positive stem cells. The EPCs expressed the endothelial markers CD34, CD31, KDR/Flk-1 and Tie-2 but also the very specific monocytic marker CD14 in different percentages of the studied cell population after 7-14 days of in vitro culture under angiogenic growth conditions. Therefore, the isolation and culture process as well as the surface markers of this EPCs indicates a different cell population from the suggested AC133/Flk-1/CD34-positive progenitor cells. But undependent of the cell source, labelled EPCs, injected into mice or rabbits with experimentally induced hind-limb ischemia, were also found to be incorporated into foci of neovascularization.[6, 19] It follows that the characterization of the phenotypic overlap between endothelial cells and these more mature hematopoietic cell

Table 1. Phenotypic analysis of putative endothelial precursor cells (modified from Schmeisser et al.[73])

Surface Antigen	Circulating Endothelial Precursors (KDR/AC133/CD34-derived)	Mature Endothelium
AC133	+	−
KDR/Flk-1	+	+
CD34	+	+
Flt-1	+	+
Flt-4	?	+[a]
VE-cadherin	+	+
vWF	+	+
CD14	−	(+)[b]
CD68	?	+
CD31 (PECAM)	+	+
CD36	?	+
Tie-2	+	+
c-kit	+	+

[a] lymphatic, tumor endothelium
[b] hepatic sinusoidal endothelium

population may help to identify their origin and to characterize the differentiation- and maturation process.

The definition of cellular phenotype traditionally relied on the expression of different surface markers. However, there are conceptual overlaps. The syncronic overlap means the consideration of two cell populations at a specific moment of time, and the comparison of their properties. The diachronic overlap describes the situation when one cell population is changing its properties while acquiring the features of another one, by a process called transdifferentiation.

3. SYNCHRONIC PHENOTYPIC OVERLAP BETWEEN MONOCYTES/ MACROPHAGES, DENDRITIC CELLS AND MATURE ENDOTHELIAL CELLS

Monocytes from the mononuclear cell fraction of peripheral blood have a high differentiation plasticity. They have the potential to give rise to macrophages or dendritic cells in response to stimulation by different cytokines and extracellular matrices.[20-22] In addition, the function and in part the phenotype of macrophages depends on the tissue in which they reside: in the lungs, for example, they differentiate in alveolar macrophages or in the sinusoide of the liver, monocytes become Kupffer cells. Interestingly, freshly isolated CD14-positive monocytes also share many surface markers with HUVECs and human microvascular endothelial cells. For example the class B scavanger receptor CD36 (microvascular ECs), CD68/macrosialin the binding protein for oxidized LDL, the adhesion molecule CD54/ICAM-1, Endoglin/CD105, CD31/PECAM-1, the VEGFR-1/Flt-1 are antigens, which are expressed by CD14-positive monocytes and ECs (HUVEC). Other surface antigens which are shared by monocytes and endothelial cells are CD40, the receptor for advanced glycation end products, RAGE and the Angiotensin receptors 1 and 2.[1, 2, 23-31] (Figure 2.).

Monocytes/macrophages and dendritic cells express HLA-DR and CD86 alone or together with CD80, which are typical markers of antigen presenting cells.[32-34] Interestingly, CD86 and HLA-DR have recently been shown also to be expressed on non-activated porcine *microvascular* ECs.[35] In addition activation leads to the additional expression of CD80 in murine cardiac ECs.[36] In human cells, Seino et al.[37] demonstrated the constitutive expression of CD86 on resting or activated HUVECs and microvascular ECs, but no CD80 expression, whereas Jollow et al.[38] reported that CD40-CD40L interactions induced the expression of CD80, but not CD86 in microvascular ECs. In contrast, Denton et al.[39] could not detect the expression of CD80 and CD86 on resting or activated HUVECs, human saphenous, vein ECs, dermal, and microvascular ECs (Figure 2.)

The CD45 family of antigens (common leucocyte antigen, LCA) is expressed by all leucocytes and plays a key role in lymphocyte activation. Forsyth et al.[40] could show the expression of the CD45RO isoform by IL-1 stimulated HUVECs. No other isoform of CD45 was detected. Leucocyte common antibodies known to detect all isoforms of CD45 did not detect endothelial CD45RO. There were clear differences in lymphocyte and endothelial CD45 molecular weight. (Fig 6,7)

3.1. In Vivo Equivalent for ECs With Phenotypical Overlap to Monocytes, Macrophages and Dendritic Cells

Indications for the in vivo existence of "hybrid" cells with endothelial and monocytic/macrophagocytic and dendritic features comes mostly from immunologic highly active tissues, such as lymphoid and hepatic tissue or inflamed atherosclerotic plaques .

Hepatic Sinusoids are highly specialized capillary vessels characterized by the presence of resident macrophages adhering to the endothelial lining. Studies in mouse embryos have shown that the specialized capillaries of the liver most likely differentiate from from capillary vessels of a mesenchymal formation, the septum transversum.[41, 42] The phenotypic characteristics of adult liver sinusoidal ECs are strikingly different from those of most other microvascular ECs of the body. Recent studies have shown that adult liver sinusoidal ECs are characterized by the constitutive expression of the following proteins: the receptors II (CD32) and III (CD16) for the Fc fragment of IgG, the lipopolysacharid-binding protein receptor (CD14) and the cell surface costimulatory signals B7-1(CD80) and B7-2 (CD86), interestingly known as classical monocyte/macrophage markers.[43-49] Another protein restricted to adult liver sinusoidal EC is the coreceptor for MHC class II molecules (CD4), a known antigen constitutively expressed on T-helper/inducer cells and monocytes/macrophages.[49] In addition, Limmer et al.[50] reported that liver sinusoidal ECs are organ-resident, non-myeloid antigen presenting cells capable of cross-presenting soluble exogenous antigens to $CD4^+$ and $CD8^+$ T cells, a feature was believed previously to be restricted to professional antigen-presenting cells such as dendritic cells. The presence of those molecules suggest that adult liver sinusoidal EC contribute to the scavenger and immune functions of hepatic sinusoids. (Figure 2.)

A further indication for an immunological function of endothelial cells was given in rejected allografts. In allograft being rejected activated microvascular endothelial cells express class II MHC molecules in vitro and in vivo, and may, therefore, provide antigen-dependent signals to CD4-positve T cells for direct activation.[51-53]

In addition, expression of the costimulatory molecule CD86 could be detected on microvascular tissue in patients with vascular neuropathy[54]. Interestingly, HLA-DR expression has also been found in aortic nonmicrovascular endothelial cells after HIV infection.[55]

Today multiple lines of evidence support the view of atherosclerosis as a chronic inflammatory disease and implicate components of the immune system in atherogenesis. The concept that intraplaque neovascularization is an important process for the progression and destabilization of atherosclerotic plaques is not new, especially since the normal intima of human arteries does not have blood vessels, these beeing confined to the adventitia and outer media.[56-59] Various functional roles have been assigned to these intimal microvessels, including the supply of nutrients and oxygen,[60] the accumulation of inflammatory blood cells, such as monocytes and T-cells within the plaques.[59] This association is also reflected by an increased expression of E-selectin, ICAM-1 and VCAM-1 in areas of plaque vascularization. Expression of these cell adhesion molecules suggest that endothelial cells lining these vessels are highly activated.[61] In addition, it has been suggested that these new blood vessels are inherently weak and therefore responsible for development of intraplaque hemorrhage, sudden increase in plaque volumen and the development of plaque instability and its consecutive cardio- and cerebrovascular complications.[62-67]

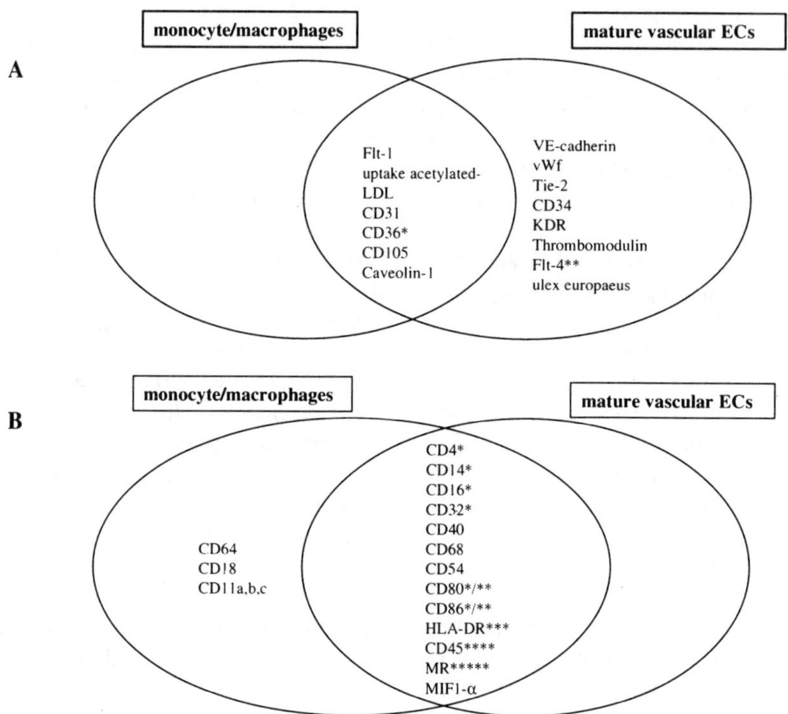

Figure 2. Schematic presentation of the synchronic phenotypic overlap between monocytes/macrophages and mature vascular endothelial cells. (**A**) Endothelial markers. (*) Microvascular ECs; (**) lymphatic endothel/HUVEC. (**B**) Leukocyte markers. (*) Hepatic sinosoidal ECs; (**) porcine microvascular ECs/controverse human data; (***) microvascular ECs/interferon-γ (IFNγ) activated HUVEC; (****) only CD45RO in IFNγ activated HUVEC; (*****) dermal microvascular ECs. (modified from Schmeisser et al.[73])

To study phenotypic features of microvascular endothelial cells within neovascularized plaque areas 42 advanced atherosclerotic plaques from 36 consecutive patients undergoing carotid endatherectomy (TEA) were examined in our laboratory. HUVECs, unstimulated and stimulated by TNF-α (10ng/ml) or VEGF (50ng/ml) were used as controls. As expected, neointimal microvessels but also HUVECs shows an intensive expression for the known endothelial marker CD34 and Tie-2. But, not expected was the uniform expression for the monocyte/macrophage marker CD68. In contrast to HUVECs or luminal macrovascular endothelial cells, intraplaque vessels stained only weak or no for von Willebrand factor (vWf). Interestingly, up to 15-20% of the microvessels stained also positive for the lipopolysacharid-binding protein receptor (CD14), the cell surface costimulatory signals B7-1(CD80) and the common leucocyte antigen CD45, known as classical monocyte/macrophage markers or leucocyte surface antigens, respectively. (Figure 3.) If these such phenotypic features of microvascular endothelial cells are only a consequence of the highly inflammatory process in the neovascularizised plaques or if they are special immunologic functions, such as antigen presentation or immune tolerance has to be clarified.

4. DIACHRONIC PHENOTYPIC OVERLAP BETWEEN MONOCYTE-DERIVED ENDOTHELIAL LIKE CELLS, DENDRITIC CELLS AND MATURE ENDOTHELIAL CELLS

Despite a lot of antigens shared by monocytes/macrophages and endothelial cells, freshly isolated CD14 positive monocytes from human peripheral blood of healthy donors do not express the classical endothelial surface markers, such as vWF, VE-cadherin, ec-NOS, Flk-1, or Tie-2. In the context of the considerable differentiation potential of monocytes/macrophages the behavior of this cell type under angiogenic (endothelial) growth conditions should be interesting.

As early as 1967 Tsapogas et al.[68] and 1972 Prathap et al.[69] postulated that intra-thrombus capillaries develop from mononuclear blood cells either already present within the clotted blood or invade the thrombus from the surrounding blood stream. Leu et al.[70] support this assumption and suggest that mononuclear cells of the mono-histiocytic system are transdifferentiated into these endothelial cells. In another experimental model, Polverini et al.[71] speculated that tumor-associated macrophages can give rise to endothelial cells.

Recently, using angiogenic culture conditions, Fernandez Pujol et al.,[72] our group[73], and Harraz et al.[74] proved that human CD14-positive monocytes, as a more differentiated hematopoietic cell type could also transdifferentiate into an endothelial-like cell type (ELC). ELCs expressed classical endothelial, mono-/macrophagocytic and dendritic markers, simultaneously. Data from our group suggest that Asahara's EPCs and the ELCs are an identical cell population, but not surprisingly, completely different to endothelial progenitor cells (positive for AC133 and/or AC133/Flk-1/CD34), described by Peichev et al.[9] and Gehling et al.[17] In particular, the initially isolated CD14 positive cells showed a typical monocyte morphology which after a few days of culture converted into adherent mononuclear cells with extended cytoplasm and small oval cells with eccentric nuclei and cytoplasmic extensions. In addition, after 6-7 days of culture, a few medium sized or large-oval cells appeared together with predominant spindle shaped cells. The cells appeared also as cell clusters comprising more round cells centrally and spindle shaped in the periphery. In the late culture multinucleated giant cells were observed.[72, 73] After 1, 2 and 4 weeks in culture the FACS-analysis, the immunocytochemical and PCR-data demonstrate a new and increasing expression for the classical endothelial cell marker vWf, VE-cadherin, ec-NOS, CD105 (Endoglin), Flt-4 and Tie-2, while the expression of the monocyte antigens CD14, CD64 decreased and for CD45 slightly decreased.[72-75] (Figure 4) Furthermore, in these cells structures resembling Weibel-Palade bodies at different storage stages were identified by electron microscopy.[72] Surprisingly, cell proliferation at low levels was stimulated by VEGF. Data remains inconsistent for the expression of the supposed stem cell (CD34) and hemangioblastic (Flk-1) markers.[52-55]

However, the simultaneous expression of CD68, CD80 (B7-1), CD86 (B7-2), HLA-DR, CD45 and CD36 indicates that ELCs might be related to macrophages. In contrast, the

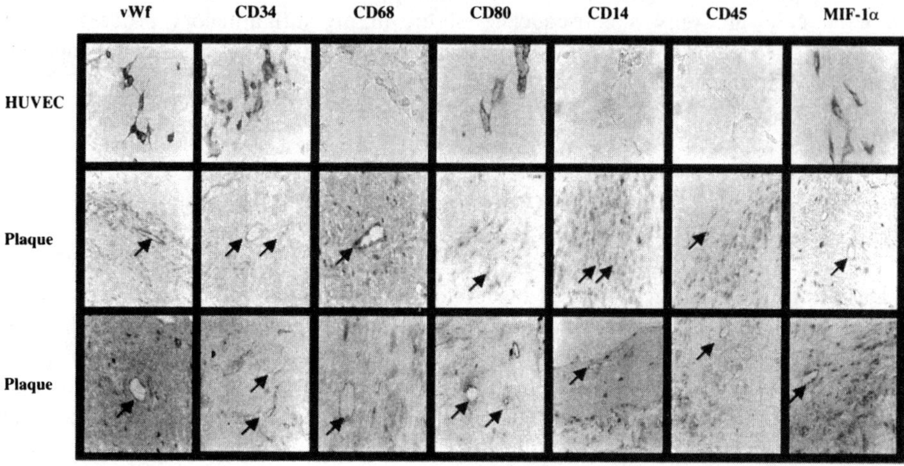

Figure 3. In Vivo Equivalent for ECs with phenotypical overlap to monocytes/macarophages. Histological examination of microvascular endothelial cells within neovascularized advanced human atherosclerotic plaques. (original magnification x 200). HUVECs, stimulated by TNF-α (10ng/ml) were used as controls. (original magnification x 100) (from Schmeisser, paper in preparation) For a color representation of this figure, see color insert at end of book.

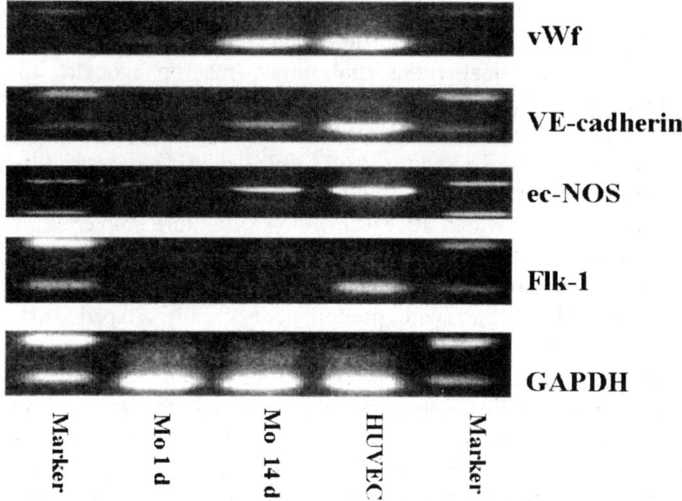

Figure 4. RT-PCR analysis of freshly isolated CD-positive monocytes after 14 days in culture with angiogenic growth factors and HUVECs. Analysed endothelial markers are vWf, VE-cadherin, ec-NOS and FLK-1. Schmeisser et al.[73]

dendritic cell (DC) markers CD1a and CD83 were not detected at any time. (summarized in Figure 5.)

Interestingly, Häusser et al.[76] showed that monocyte-derived immature DCs maintain their ability to differentiate into macrophages and thus represent an intermediate differentiation stage. However, Fernandez Pujol et al.[75] presented data, that monocyte-derived immature DCs (CD1a, HLA-DR and CD86 positive), propagated with GM-CSF and IL-4, showed a weak, but significant expression of the endothelial cell markers vWF, VE-cadherin, Flt-1 and Flt-4. Maturation of DCs, induced by TNF-α, resulted in a typical morphology with extended dendrites, upregulation of T-cell costimulatory molecules (CD80, CD86), appearance of the maturation marker CD83, increase of MHC class II expression and a strong capacity to prime naive T-cells.[77, 78] The signals of vWf and VE-cadherin remained unchanged or increased only slightly.

On the other hand, when immature DCs were cultured in the presence of angiogenic growth factors including VEGF, Oncostatin and IL-4 the cultured cells developed into ELCs, characterized by an increased expression of the endothelial markers together with a disappearance of the dendritic markers CD1a and CD83. In mixed lymphocyte cultures ELCs derived from immature DCs exhibited only a moderate stimulation of allogenic T cells. Mature DCs were more potent APCs than ELCs in this experimental model, whereas HUVECs showed no antigen presenting features.[75] In this respect, the angiogenic growth factor VEGF could have a great significance. Findings of Gabrilovich et al.,[79] Oyama et al.,[80] and Ohm et al.[81] showed, that VEGF causes a defect in the maturation of DCs from progenitors. They suggested that VEGF activation of the VEGFR-1 (Flt-1) is able to block the Flt-3-ligand induced activation of NF-κB, a mechanism associated with the functional maturation of DCs.

Thus, the results indicate that not only CD14-positive monocytes have a multilineage potential of differentiation in the presence of specific cytokines, but also immature dendritic cells derived from peripheral CD14-positive monocytes which could transdifferentiate into macrophages and ELCs. (Figure 6.)

Regarding these results, it would be interesting to determine if the induction of VE-cadherin, vWF and other endothelial markers in these hematopoietic cells is associated with the induction of the regulating transcriptional factors, which have been identified for these molecules in endothelial cells. Similarly the role of these transcription factors, which regulate as far as is known the specific differentiation and maturation of the monocyte/macrophage transition (e.g. SCL, PU.1, EGR-1, HOXB7) as well as endothelial cell development (e.g. SCL, GATA-2, c-Ets1, HIF-2α), remains to be elucidated this specific transdifferentiation process.[1, 82-84]

4.1. In Vivo Equivalent for Monocyte-Derived ELCs

So far, solid evidences for the in vivo existence of monocyte-derived ELCs was not provided. Some data indicate that cells lining human lymph node sinuses and splenic sinusoids represent a special subset of macrophages with endothelial cell features. They express antigens that are associated with monocyte/macrophages and ECs.[85-86]

Whether Kaposi's sarcoma is a true neoplasm or a reactive endothelial cell outgrowth triggered by inflammatory cytokines remains unclear. The spindle shaped cells (KS cells), the histological hallmark of the disease, and peripheral blood derived KS-like

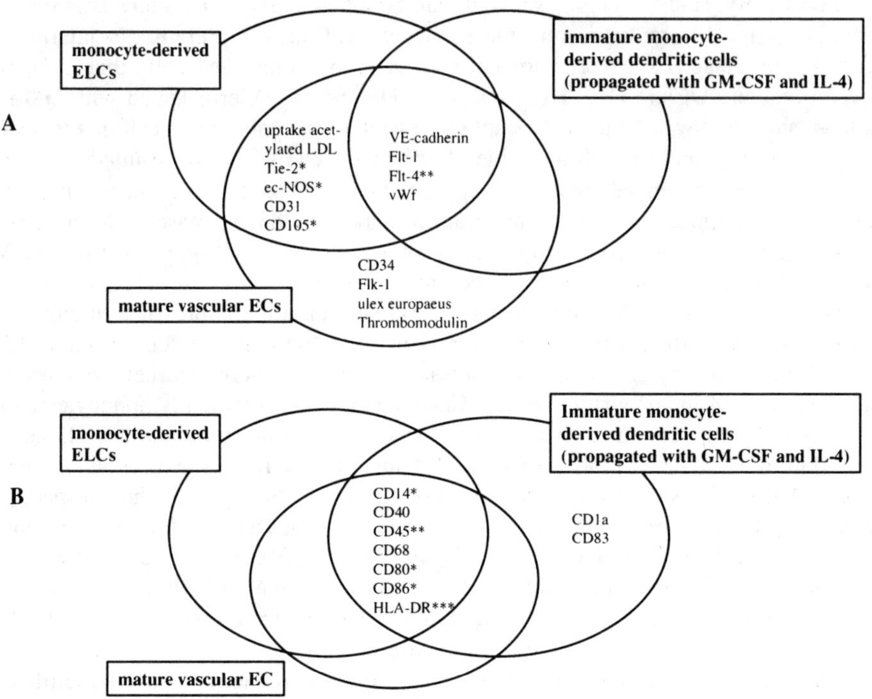

Figure 5. Schematic presentation of the diachronic phenotypic overlap between monocyte-derived ELCs, immature monocyte-derived DCs, and mature vascular endothelial cells. (A) Endothelial markers. (*) No data in DCs; (**) mature vascular Ecs, lymphatic and tumor endothelium. (B) Leukocyte markers. (*) Hepatic sinosoidal ECs; (**) only CD45RO in IFN-γ-acivated HUVECs; (***) microvascular ECs/interferon-γ (IFNγ) activated HUVECs.(modified from Schmeisser et al.[73])

cells are characterized by coexpression of macrophage and endothelial antigens CD45, CD68, mannose receptor, CD14, Ve-cadherin, vWF, Flk-1 and Flt-4. Uccini et al.[87] suggested that KS-lesions derive from tissue accumulation and local proliferation of a special subset of macrophages with endothelial features. In contrast, the high expression of KDR and Flt-4 by KS-cells argue in favour a vascular origin, specifically from lymphatic endothelium.[88-89]

In different experimental models for ischemia it was shown that EPCs[5] or CD14-positive monocytes (ELCs) together with CD34 enriched progenitor cells[74] incorporate into foci of neovascularization, after these cells have been expanded in vitro. It remains to be resolved if the labelled EPCs or ELCs in these foci represent vascular cells installed into host capillaries or monocyte/macrophages traversing the endothelium. In fact, blood flow recovery and capillary density in the different ischemic regions were markedly

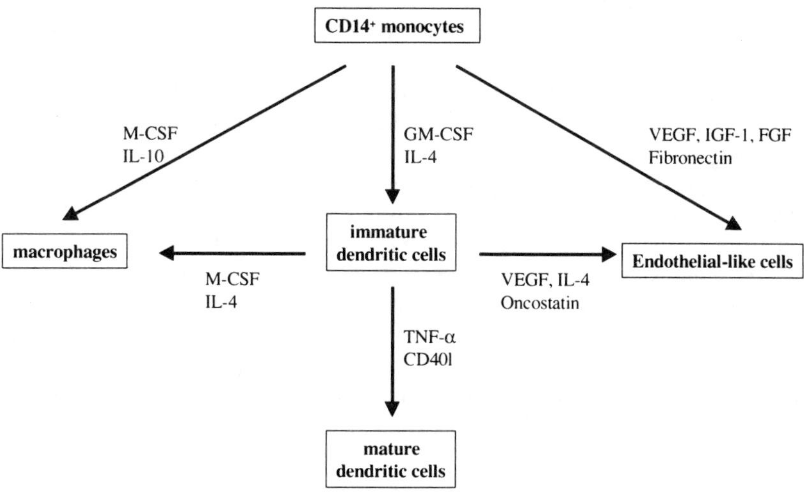

Figure 6. Hypothesis of a multilineage capacity by CD14-positive monocytes in the presence of specific cytokines. (Schmeisser et al.[73])

improved by these activated cells, which might be also simply the result of angiogenic growth factor secretion by the used mononuclear cell population.[90]

Recently, Moldovan et al.[91] published an interesting study that could lead to a shift in our thinking on the mechanism of neovascularization in ischemic tissues. Already, in vitro data indicate that monocyte-derived endothelial like cells have the potential to form cord- and tubular like structures in vitro.[72-75] In combination with the formation of VE-cadherin as a cell-cell contact signal, the structures might represent the preformation of vascular lines. In fact, Moldovan et al. demonstrated in vivo findings in transgenic mice, overexpressing MCP-1, that invading macrophages drill an extensive network of tunnels within the ischemic heart. Most interestingly, many of the tunnels seem to contain erythrocytes. In this context, known data, such as macrophage activities within hypoxic and necrotic tumor areas promote angiogenesis, tumor growth and metastasis appear in a new light.[92, 93] It remains to be elucidated, if there exist a morphological correlation in conditions of pathological angiogenesis for this possible direct role of monocyte/macrophages in neovascularization processes.

5. CONCLUSIONS

Phenotypic analysis shows that the monocyte/macrophage/dendritic cell system is closely related to endothelial cells. This holds specifically true for the endothelial cells derived from sinusoidal and microvascular endothelial cells. Comparative studies of morphological and surface antigen expression markers indicate that monocytes or monocyte precursors or immature DCs, depending on the local angiogenic growth conditions, may differentiate into endothelial like cells (ELCs) and, moreover, form cord- and tubular-like structures in vitro. In MCP-1 overexpressing transgenic mice an endothelium-independent revascularization potential by macrophages, which form "tunnel-like structures" in ischemic regions, was also suggested. Future studies should address the question, whether ELCs develop a similar functional behaviour in vasoregulation, coagulation and fibrinolysis, such as described in vascular ECs.

So far, a definitive proof for an angioblastic and revascularizising "tunnel-forming" potential of monocytes was not provided. Such potential of monocytes would be of fundamental research interest and certainly would sprout extensive research activities focussing on transdifferentiation capability of somewhat more differentiated cells such as monocytes and dendritic cells.

6. REFERENCES

1. C. Garlanda, and E. Dejana, Heterogenity of endothelial cells. Specific markers, *Arterioscler Tromb Vasc Biol.* **17**, 1193-1202 (1997).
2. D. B. Cines, ES. Pollak, C. A. Buck, J. Loscalzo, G. A. Zimmermann, R. P. McEver, J. S. Pober, T. M. Wick, B. A. Konkle, B. S. Schwatz, E. S. Barnathan, K. R. McCrae, B. A. Hug, A. M. Schmidt, and D. Stern, Endothelial cells in physiology and in the pathophysiology of vascular disorders, *Blood* **91**, 3527-3561 (1997).
3. T. N. Sato, Y. Qin, C. A. Kozak, and KL Audus, Tie-1 and Tie-2 define another class of putative receptor tyrosine kinase genes expressed in early embryonic vascular system, (erratum 1993, 90:12056), *Proc Natl Acad Sci* (USA) **90**, 9355-9358 (1993).
4. F. Shalaby, J. Ho, W. L. Stanford, K. D. Fischer, A. C. Schuh, L. Schwartz, A. Bernstein and J. Rossant, A requirement for Flk-1 in primitive and definitive hematopoiesis and vasculogenesis, *Cell* **89**, 981-990 (1999).
5. A. Eichmann, C. Corbel, V. Nataf, P. Vaigot, C. Breant, and N. M. L. Douarin, Ligand-dependent development of the endothelial and hemopoietic lineages from embryonic mesodermal cells expressing vascular endothelial growth factor receptor 2, *Proc Natl Acad Sci* (USA) **94**, 5141-5146 (1997).
6. T. Asahara, T. Murohara, A. Sullivan, M. Silver, R. van der Zee, T. Li, B. Witzenbichler, G. Schattemann , and J. M. Isner, Isolation of putative progenitor endothelial cells for angiogenesis, *Science* **275**, 964-967 (1997).
7. M. Nieda, A. Nicol, P. Denning-Kendall, J. Sweetenham, B. Bradle, and J. Hows, Endothelial cell precursors are normal components of human umbilical cord blood, *British J Haematology* **98**, 775-777 (1997).
8. B. Q. Shi, S. Rafii, M. H. D. Wu, E. S. Wijelath, C. Yu, A. Ishida, Y. Fujita, S. Kothari, R. Mohle, L. R. Sauvage, M. A. S. Moore, R. F. Storb, and W. P. Hammond, Evidence for circulating bone marrow-derived endothelial cells, *Blood* **92**, 362-367 (1998).
9. M. Peichev, A. J. Naiyer, D. Pereira, Z. Zhu, W. J. Lane, M. Williams, M. C. Oz, D. J. Hicklin, L. Witte, M. S. Moore, and S. Rafii, Expression of VEGFR-2 and AC133 by circulating human CD34$^+$ cells identifies a population of functional endothelial precursors, *Blood* **95**, 952-958 (2000).
10. T. Mustonen, and K. Alitalo, Endothelial receptor tyrosine kinases involved in angiogenesis, *J Cell Biol* **129**, 895-902 (1995).
11. F. Shalaby, J. Rossant, T. P. Yamaguchi, M. Gertsenstein, X. F. Wu, M. L. Breitman, and A. C. Schuh, Failure of blood island formation and vasculogenesis in Flk-1-deficient mice, *Nature* **376**, 62-66 (1995).

12. J. Yamashita, H. Itoh, M. Hirashima, M. Ogawa, S. Nishikawa, T. Yurugi, M. Naito, K. Nakao, and S. I. Nishikawa, Flk1-positive cells derived from embryonic stem cells serve as vascular progenitors, *Nature* **408**, 92-96 (2000).

13. B. L. Ziegler, M. Valtieri, G. A. Porada, R. De Maria, R. Muller, B. Masella, M. Gabbianelli, I. Casella, E. Pelosi, T. Bock, E. D. Zanjani, and C. Peschle, KDR receptor: a key marker defining hematopoietic stem cells, *Science* **285**, 1553-1558 (1999).

14. K. Choi, M. Kennedy, A. Kazarow, J. C. Papadimitiou, and G. Keller, A common precursor for hematopoietic and endothelial cells, *Development* **125**, 725-732 (1998).

15. S. Miraglia, W. Godfrey, A. H. Yin, K. Atkins, R .Warnke, J. T. Holden, R. A. Bray, E. K. Waller, and D. W. Buck, A novel five-transmembrane hematopoietic stem cell antigen: isolation, characterization, and molecular cloning, *Blood* **90**, 5013-5021 (1997).

16. A. H. Yin, S. Miraglia, E. D. Zaniani, G. Almeida-Porada, M. Ogawa, A. G. Leary, J. Olweus, J. Kearney, and D. W. Buck, AC133, a novel marker for human hematopoietic stem and progenitor cells, *Blood* **90**, 5002-5012 (1997).

17. U. M.Gehling, S. Ergün, U. Schumacher, C. Wagener, K. Pantel, M. Otte, G. Schuch, P. Schaffhausen, T. Mende, N. Kilic, K. Kluge, B. Schäfer, D. K. Hossfeld, and W. Fiedler, In vitro differentiation of endothelial cells from AC133-positive progenitor cells, *Blood* **95**, 3106-3112 (2000).

18. T. Asahara, H. Masuda, T. Takahashi, C. Kalka, C. Pastore, M. Silver, M. Kearne, M. Magner, and J. M. Isner, Bone marrow origin of endothelial progenitor cells responsible for postnatal Vasculogenesis in physiological and pathological neovascularization, *Circ Res* **85**, 221-228 (1999).

19. C. Kalka, H. Masuda, T. Takahashi, M. Kalka-Moll, M. Silver, M. Kearney, T. Li, J. M. Isner, and T. Asahara, Transplantation of ex vivo expanded endothelial progenitor cells for therapeutic Neovascularization, *Proc Natl Acad Sci* (USA) **97**, 3422-3427 (2000).

20. M. Shima, S. L. Teitelbaum, V. M. Holers, C. Ruzicka, P. Osmack, and F. P. Ross, Macrophage-colony-stimulating factor regulates expression of the integrins alpha 4 beta 1 and alpha 5 beta 1 by murine bone marrow macrophages, *Proc Natl Acad Sci* (USA) **92**, 5179-5183 (1995).

21. R. Giavazzi, and I. R. Hart, Mononuclear phagocyte adherence in the presence of laminin. A possible marker of cellular differentiation, *Exp Cell Res* **146**, 391-399 (1993).

22. J. M. Austin, and D. Phil, Dendritic cells, *Curr Opin Hematol* **5**, 3-15 (1998).

23. C. Trezzini, T. W. Jungi, M. O. Spycher, F. E. Maly, and P. Rao, Human monocytes CD36 and CD16 are signaling molecules. Evidence from studies using antibody-induced chemiluminescence as a tool to probe signal transduction, *Immunology* **71**, 29-37 (1990).

24. H. Strobl, C. Scheinecker, B. Cesmarits, O. Majdic, and W. Knapp, Flow cytometric analysis of intracellular CD68 molecule expression in normal and malignant heamapoiesis, *British J Haematol.* **90**, 774-782 (1995).

25. G. Ocklind, D. Friedrichs, and J. H. Peters, Expression of CD54, CD58, CD14,, and HLA-DR on macrophage and macrophage derived accessory cells and their accessory capacity, *Immunol Lett* **31**, 253-258 (1992).

26. S. H. Lee, P. R. Crocker, S. Westaby, N. Key, D. Y. Mason, S. Gordon, and D. J. Weatherall, Isolation and immunocytochemical characterization of human bone marrow stromal macrophages in hemopoietic clusters, *J Exp Med* **168**, 1193-1198 (1988).

27. P. J. Newman, and S. M. Albelda, Cellular and molecular aspects of PECAM-1, *Nouv Rev Fr Hematol* **34**, Suppl:S9-13 (1992).

28. A. Sawano, S. Iwai, Y. Sakurai, M. Ito, K. Shitara, T. Nakahata, and M. Shibuya, Flt-1, vascular endothelial growth factor receptor 1, is a novel cell surface marker for the lineage of monocyte-macrophages in humans, *Blood* **97**, 785-791(2001).

29. A. M. Schmidt, S. D. Yan, J. Brett, R. Mora, R. Nowygrod, and D. Stern, Regulation of human mononuclear phagocyte migration by cell surface-binding proteins for advanced glycation end products, *J Clin Invest* **91**, 2155-2168 (1993).

30. J. Banchereau, F. Bazan, D. Blanchard, F. Briere, J. P. Galizzi, C. van Kooten, Y. J. Liu, F. Rousset, and S. Sealand, The CD40 antigen and ist ligand, *Annu Rev Immunol* **12**, 881-922 (1994).

31. K. Shimada, and Y. Yazaki, Binding sites for angiotensin II in human leucocytes, *J Biochem* **84**, 1013-1015 (1978).

32. C. L. Manyak, H. Tse, P. Fischer, L. Coker, N. H. Signal, and G. C. Koo, Regulation of class II MHC molecules on human endothelial cells. Effects of IFN and dexamethasone, *J Immunol* **140**, 3817-3822 (1988).

33. A. Shore, P. Leary, and J. M. Teitel, Comparison of accessory cell functions of endothelial cells and monocytes: Il-2 production by T cells and PFC generation, *Cell Immunol* **100**, 210-217 (1986).

34. P. H. Hart, G. A. Whitty, D. R. Burgess, M. Croatto, and J. A. Hamilton, Augmentation of glucocorticoid action on human monocytes by interleucin-4, *Lymphokine Res* **9**, 147-153 (1990).

35. I. Vallee, J. M. Guillaumin, G. Thibault, Y. Gruel, Y. Lebranchu, P. Bardos, and H. Watier, Human T lymphocyte proliferative response to resting porcine endothelial cells results from an HLA-restricted, IL-10 sensitive, indirect presentation pathway but also depends on endothelial-specific costimulatory factors, *J Immunol* **161**, 1652-1658 (1998).

36. W. W. Hancock, M. H. Sayegh, X. G. Zheng, R. Peach, and P. S. Linsley, Costimulatory function and expression of CD40 ligand, CD80, and CD86 in vascularized murine cardiac allograft rejection, *Proc Natl Acad Sci* (USA) **93**, 13967-13973 (1996).

37. K. Seino, M. Azuma, H. Bashuda, K. Fukao, H. Yagita, and K. Okumura, CD86 (B70/B7-2) on endothelial cells co-stimulates allogeneic CD4+ T cells, *Int Immunol* **7**, 1331-1337 (1995).

38. K. C. Jollow, J. C. Zimring, J.B. Sundstrom, and A. A. Ansari, CD40 ligation induced phenotypic and functional expression of CD80 by human cardiac microvascular endothelial cells, *Transplantation* **68**, 430-439 (1999).

39. M.D. Dentn, C. S. Geehan, S. I. Alexander, M. H. Sayegh, and D. M. Briscoe, Endothelial cells modify the costimulatory capacity of transmigrating leukocytes and promote CD28-mediated CD4(+) T cell alloactivation, *J Exp Med* **190**, 555-566 (1999).

40. K. D. Forsyth, K. Y. Chua, V. Talbot, and W. R. Thomas, Expression of the Leucocyte Common Antigen CD45 by endothelium, *J Immunol* **150**, 3471-3477 (1993).

41. V. Desmet, Embryology of the liver and intrahepatic biliary tract, and an overview of malformations of the bile duct. In: *Oxford Textbook of Clinical Hepatology*, edited by N. McIntyre, J. P. Benhamou, J. Bircher and J. Rodes, (Oxford, UK Oxford,1991), pp. 497

42. G. Machiarelli, S. Makabe, and P. Motta, Scanning electron microscopy of adult and fetal liver sinusoids, In: *Sinusoids in Human Liver: Health and Disease*, edited by P. Biolac-Sage, and C. Balabaud, (Rijswijk, The Netherlands, Kupfer Cell Foundation, 1988) pp.63

43. Steinhoff G, M Behrend, B Schrader, AM Duijvestijn and K Wonigeit, Expression patterns of leukocyte adhesion ligand molecules on human liver endothelia. Lack of ELAM-1 and CD62 inducibility on sinusoidal endothelia and distinct distribution of VCAM-1, ICAM-1, ICAM-2, and LFA-3, *Am J Pathol* **142**, 481-488 (1993).

44. M. Garcia-Barcina, B. Lukomska, W. Gawron, M. Winnock, F. Vidal-Vanaclocha, P. Bioulac-Sage, C. Balabaud, and W. Olszewski, Expression of cell adhesion molecules on liver-associated lymphocytes and their ligands on sinusoidal lining cells in patients with benign or malignant liver disease, *Am J Pathol* **146**, 1406-1413 (1995).

45. A. W. Lohse, P. A. Knolle, K. Bilo, A. Uhrig, C. Waldmann, M. Ibe, E. Schmitt, G. Gerken, and K. H. Meyer Zum Buschenfelde, Antigen-presenting function and B7 expression of murine sinusoidal endothelial cells and Kupffer cells, *Gastroenterology* **110**, 1175-1181(1996).

46. P. A. Knolle, A. Uhrig, S. Hegenbarth, E. Loser, E. Schmitt, G. Gerken, and A. W. Lohse, IL-10 down-regulates T cell activation by antigen-presenting liver sinusoidal endothelial cells through decreased antigen uptake via the mannose receptor and lowered surface expression of accessory molecules, *Clin Exp Immunol* **114**, 427-433 (1998).

47. P. A. Knolle, and G. Gerken, Local control of the immune response in the liver, *Immunol Rev* **174**, 21-34 (2000).

48. P. A. Knolle, and A. Limmer, Neighborhood politics: the immunoregulatory function of organ-resident liver endothelial cells, *Trends Immunol* **22**, 432-437 (2001).

49. J. Y. Scoazec, and G. Feldmann, In situ immunophenotyping study of endothelial cells of the human hepatic sinusoid: results and functional implications, *Hepatology* **14**, 789-797 (1991).

50. A. Limmer, J. Ohl, C. Kurts, H. G. Ljunggren, Y. Reiss, M. Groettrup, F. Momburg, B. Arnold, and P. A. Knolle, Efficient presentation of exogenous antigen by liver endothelial cells to CD8+ T cells results in antigen-specific T-cell tolerance, *Nat Med* **6**, 348-1354 (2000).

51. C. Page, M. Rose, M. Yacoub, and R. Pigott, Antigenic heterogeneity of vascular endothelium, *Am J Pathol* **141**, 673-683 (1992).

52. D. M. Briscoe, L. E. DesRoches, J. M. Kiely, J. A. Lederer, and A. H. Lichtman, Antigen-dependent activation of T helper cell subsets by endothelium, *Transplantation* **59**, 1638-1641 (1995).

53. D. M. Briscoe, P. Ganz, S. I. Alexander, R. J. Melder, R. K. Jain, R. S. Cotran, and A. H. Lichtman, The problem of chronic rejection: influence of leukocyte-endothelial interactions, *Kidney Int Suppl* **58**, S22-27 (1997).

54. I. Van Rhijn, L. H. Van den Berg, W. M. Bosboom, H. G. Otten, and T. Logtenberg, Expression of accessory molecules for T-cell activation in peripheral nerve of patients with CIDP and vasculitic neuropathy, *Brain* **123**, 2020-2029 (2000).

55. C. Zietz, B. Hotz, M. Sturzl, E. Rauch, R. Penning, and U. Lohrs, Aortic endothelium in HIV-1 infection: chronic injury, activation, and increased leukocyte adherence, *Am J Pathol* **149**, 1887-1898 (1996).

56. W. Koster, Endarteritis and arteritis, *Berl Klin Wochenschr* **13**, 454-57 (1876).

57. N. Kumamoto, Y. Nakashima, K. Suieshi, Intimal neovascularization in human coronary atherosclerosis: its origin and pathophysiological significance, *Hum Pathol* **26**, 450-56 (1995).
58. E. O'Brien, M. R. Garwin, R. Dev, D. K. Stewart, T. Hinohara, J. B. Simpson, and S. M. Schwartz, Angiogenesis in human coronary atherosclerotic plaques, *Am J Pathol* **145**, 883-93 (1994).
59. Y. Zhang, W. J. Cliff, G. I. Schoefl, and G.Higgins, Immunohistochemical study of intimal microvessels in coronary atherosclerosis, *Am J Pathol.* **143**, 164-172 (1993)
60. E. Groszek, and S. M. Grundy, The possible role of the arterial microcirculation in the pathogenesis of atherosclerosis, *J Chron Dis* **33**, 679-684 (1980)
61. K. D. O'Brien, T. O. McDonald, A. Chait, M. D. Allen, C. E. Alpers, Neovascular expression of E-selectin, intercellular adhesion molecule-1, and vascular cell adhesion molecule-1 in human atherosclerosis and their relation to intimal leucocyte content, *Circulation* **93**, 672-82 (1996).
62. A. C. Barger, R. Beeuwkes, L. L. Lainey et al, Vasa vasorum aand neovascularization of human coronary arteries: a possible role in the pathophysiology of atherosclerosis, *N Eng J Med* **310**, 175-177 (1984).
63. J. A. Fryer, P. C. Myers, and M. Appleberg, Carotid intraplaque heamorrhage: the significance of neovascularity, *J Vasc Surg* **6**, 341-9 (1987).
64. M. Jeziorska, and D. E. Wooley, Local neovascularization and cellular composition within vulnerable regions of atherosclerotic plaques of human carotid arteries, *J Pathol.* **188,** 189-196 (1999).
65. A. N. Tenaglia, A. G. Peters, M. H. Sketch, and B. H. Annex, Neovascularization in atherectomy specimens from patients with unstable angina:implications for pathogenesis of unstable angina, *Am Heart J* **135**, 10-14 (1998).
66. M. J. Mc Carthy, I. M. Loftus, M. M. Thompson, I. Jones, N. J. M. London, P. R. F. Bell, R. Naylor, and N. P. J. Prindle, Angiogenesis and the atherosclerootic carotid plaque: an association between symptomatology and plaque morphology, *J Vasc Surg* **22**, 261-8 (1999).
67. M. Jeziorska, and D. E. Wooley, Local neovascularization and cellular composition within vulnerable regions of atherosclerotic plaques of human carotid arteries, *J Pathol* **188**, 189-196 (1999).
68. M. J. Tsapogas, G. A. Streling, and M. B. Girolami, Study on the organization of experimental thrombi, *Angiology* **18**, 825-832 (1967).
69. K. Prathap, Surface lining cells of healing thrombi in rat femoral veins, an electron-microscopic study, *J Pathol* **107**, 1-8 (1972).
70. H. J. Leu, W. Feigl, and M. Susani, Angiogenesis from mononuclear cells in thrombi, *Virchows Arch A* **411**, 5-14 (1987).
71. P. J. Polverini, and S. J. Leibovich, Induction of neovascularization in vivo and endothelial proliferation in vitro by tumor-associated macrophages, *Lab Invest* **51**, 635-642 (1984).
72. B. Fernandez Pujol, F. C. Lucibello, U. M. Gehling, K. Lindemann, N. Weidner, M. L. Zuzarte, J. Adamkiewicz, II. P. Elsasser, R. Muller, and K. Havemann, Endothelial-like cells derived from human CD14 positive monocytes, *Differentiation* **65**, 287-300 (2000).
73. A. Schmeisser, C. D. Garlichs, H. Zhang, S. Eskafi, C. Graffy, J. Ludwig, R. H. Strasser, and W. G. Daniel, Monocytes coexpress endothelial and macrophagocytic lineage markers and form cord-like structures in Matrigel under angiogenic conditions, *Cardiovasc Res* **49**, 671-680 (2001).
74. M. Harraz, C. Jiao, H. D. Hanlon, R. S. Hartley, and G. C. Schatteman, Cd34(-) blood-derived human endothelial cell progenitors, *Stem Cells* **19**, 304-312 (2001).
75. B. Fernandez Pujol, F. C. Lucibello, M. Zuzarte, P. Lutjens, R. Muller, and K. Havemann, Dendritic cells derived from peripheral monocytes express endothelial markers and in the presence of angiogenic growth factors differentiate into endothelial-like cells, *Eur J Cell Biol* **80**, 99-110 (2001).
76. G. Hausser, B. Ludewig, H. R. Gelderblom, Y. Tsunetsugu-Yokota, K. Akagawa, and A. Meyerhans, Monocyte-derived dendritic cells represent a transient stage of differentiation in the myeloid lineage, *Immunobiology* **5**, 534-542 (1997).
77. F. Sallusto, and A. Lanzavecchia, Efficient presentation of soluble antigen by cultured human dendritic cells is maintained by granulocyte/macrophage colony-stimulating factor plus interleukin 4 and downregulated by tumor necrosis factor alpha, *J Exp Med* **4**, 1109-1118 (1994).
78. L. J. Zhou, and T. F. Tedder, CD14+ blood monocytes can differentiate into functionally mature CD83+ dendritic cells, *Proc Natl Acad Sci* (U S A) **93**, 2588-2592 (1996).
79. D. I. Gabrilovich, H. L. Chen, K. R. Girgis, H. T. Cunningham, G. M. Meny, S. Nadaf, D. Kavanaugh, and D. P. Carbone, Production of vascular endothelial growth factor by human tumors inhibits the functional maturation of dendritic cells, *Nat Med* **10**, 1096-1103. (1996).
80. T. Oyama, S. Ran, T. Ishida, S. Nadaf, L. Kerr, D. P. Carbone, and D. I. Gabrilovich, Vascular endothelial growth factor affects dendritic cell maturation through the inhibition of nuclear factor-kappa B activation in hemopoietic progenitor cells, *J Immunol* **160**, 1224-1232 (1998).
81. J. E. Ohm, M. R. Shurin, C. Esche, M. T. Lotze, D. P. Carbone, and D. I. Gabrilovich, Effect of vascular

endothelial growth factor and FLT3 ligand on dendritic cell generation in vivo, *J Immunol* **163**, 3260-3268 (1999).

82. A. F. Valledor, F. E. Borras, M. Cullell-Young, and A. Celada, Transcription factors that regulate monocyte/macrophage differentiation, *J Leukoc Biol* **63**, 405-417 (1998).

83. A. Kappel, V. Ronicke, A. Damert, I. Flamme, W. Risau, and G. Breier, Identification of vascular endothelial growth factor (VEGF) receptor-2 (Flk-1) promoter/enhancer sequences sufficient for angioblast and endothelial cell-specific transcription in transgenic mice, *Blood* **93**, 4284-4292 (1999).

84. A. Kappel, T. M. Schlaeger, I. Flamme, S. H. Orkin, W. Risau, and G. Breier, Role of SCL/Tal-1, GATA, and ets transcription factor binding sites for the regulation of flk-1 expression during murine vascular development, *Blood* **96**, 3078-3085 (2000).

85. C. D. Baroni, D. Vitolo, D. Remotti, A. Biondi, F. Pezzella, L. P. Ruco, and S. Uccini, Immunohistochemical heterogeneity of macrophage subpopulations in human lymphoid tissues, *Histopathology* **11**, 1029-1042 (1987).

86. P. J. Buckley, S. A. Dickson, and W. S. Walker, Human splenic sinusoidal lining cells express antigens associated with monocytes, macrophages, endothelial cells, and T lymphocytes, *J Immunol* **134**, 2310-2315 (1985).

87. S. Uccini, M. C. Sirianni, L. Vincenzi, S. Topino, A. Stoppacciaro, I. Lesnoni La Parola, M. Capuano, C. Masini, D. Cerimele, M. Cella, A. Lanzavecchia, P. Allavena, A. Mantovani, C. D. Baroni, and L. P. Ruco, Kaposi's sarcoma cells express the macrophage-associated antigen mannose receptor and develop in peripheral blood cultures of Kaposi's sarcoma patients, *Am J Pathol* **150**, 929-938 (1997).

88. M. Skobe, L. F. Brown, K. Tognazzi, R. K. Ganju, B. J. Dezube, K. Alitalo, and M. Detmar, Vascular endothelial growth factor-C (VEGF-C) and its receptors KDR and flt-4 are expressed in AIDS-associated Kaposi's sarcoma, *J Invest Dermatol* **113**, 1047-1053 (1999).

89. S. Marchio, L. Primo, M. Pagano, G. Palestro, A. Albini, T. Veikkola, I. Cascone, K. Alitalo, and F. Bussolino, Vascular endothelial growth factor-C stimulates the migration and proliferation of Kaposi's sarcoma cells, *J Biol Chem* **274**, 27617-27622 (1999).

90. W. Schaper, and W. D. Ito, Molecular mechanisms of coronary collateral vessel growth, Circ Res **79**, 911-919 (1996).

91. N. I. Moldovan, P. J. Goldschmidt-Clermont, J. Parker-Thornburg, S. D. Shapiro, and P. E. Kolattukudy, Contribution of monocytes/macrophages to compensatory neovascularization: the drilling of metalloelastase-positive tunnels in ischemic myocardium, *Circ Res* **87**, 378-384. (2000).

92. R. D. Leek, C. E. Lewis, R. Whitehouse, M. Greenall, J. Clarke, and A. L. Harris, Association of macrophage infiltration with angiogenesis and prognosis in invasive breast carcinoma, *Cancer Res* **56**, 4625-4629 (1996).

93. R. D. Leek, R. J. Landers, A. L. Harris, and C. E. Lewis, Necrosis correlates with high vascular density and focal macrophage infiltration in invasive carcinoma of the breast, *Br J Cancer* **79**, 991-995 (1999).

DISSECTION OF MONOCYTE AND ENDOTHELIAL ACTIVITIES BY USING VEGF-RECEPTOR SPECIFIC LIGANDS

Matthias Clauss[*], Frederic Pipp[*], Katja Issbrücker[*], Herbert Weich[+], Matthias Heil[*], and Wolfgang Schaper[*]

1. DIVERSE ACTIVITIES OF VEGF

Vascular endothelial growth factor (VEGF) is the major inducer of angiogenesis and vasculogenesis (Risau, 1997). It was isolated based on its ability to induce proliferation of endothelial cells but not fibroblasts (Leung et al., 1989). Based on this competency VEGF emerged as a highly good candidate as an angiogenesis-specific factor. Because VEGF is produced in response to hypoxia it describes a physiological mean to ablate the need of nutrients and oxygen by the induction of new blood vessels. In vitro, it induces several activities in endothelial cells, which are believed to be associated with angiogenesis, such as proliferation, survival and migration. But it also displays activities in endothelial cells, which were different from what was expected from an endothelial cell specific mitogen. VEGF can also induce vascular hyperpermeability, leading to its original description as vascular permeability factor (VPF) and turned out to be an inducer of tissue factor, the initiator of blood coagulation (Nemerson, 1988) . In addition it is able to increase both the plasminogen activator and its inhibitor (Pepper et al., 1991). VEGF was found to cause release of von Willebrand factor from the Weibel-Palade bodies in endothelial cells and to increase the surface expression of P-selectin, two processes which comprise possible links to blood coagulation and inflammation, respectively. In consequence, the question arose whether VEGF would be a jack of all trades, comparable to another unspecific growth factor, fibroblast growth factor (FGF) (Clauss and Schaper, 2000). This point of view was enforced by the early finding that VEGF not only acts on endothelial cells but also on other cells. In this context monocytes were identified shortly after the discovery of VEGF as vascular endothelial growth factor (Clauss et al., 1990). In monocytes, VEGF induces chemotaxis, transmigration through endothelial monolayers, tissue factor and the inducible NO-Synthetase (Clauss, 1998). Furthermore, it was found to inhibit the differentiation to dendritic cells and to enforce the transition to endothelial cells (Gabrilovich et al., 1998). These diverse activities are not necessarily

[*]Max-Planck-Institute for Physiological & Clinical Research, Bad Nauheim, D-61231 and the German Research Center for Biotechnology (GBF), Braunschweig, D-38124[+]

Novel Angiogenic Mechanisms: Role of Circulating Progenitor Endothelial Cells.
Edited by Nicanor I. Moldovan, Kluwer Academic/Plenum Publishers, 2003.

associated with angiogenesis. It should therefore be important to understand the mechanism of VEGF-elicited activities and, if possible to be able to distinguish VEGF-mediated activities on endothelial cells from those onto monocytes.

2. DIFFERENTIAL VEGF-RECEPTOR EXPRESSION ON MONOCYTES AND ENDOTHELIAL CELLS

A first clue to the diverse action of VEGF on endothelial cells and monocytes arose from comparison of the receptor expression these cells. In contrast to endothelial cells, which express both VEGF receptors, cells of the monocyte/macrophage lineage exhibit only one specific binding site (Shen et al. 1993). This binding site was identified as Flt-1 (designated as VEGFR-1) by means of Northern blotting analysis and PCR-studies (Barleon et al. 1996; Clauss et al. 1996). Based on the ability of VEGF to induce numerous biological activities in mononuclear phagocytes, Flt-1 was demonstrated as a functional receptor for monocytes and macrophages. When placental growth factor (PlGF) in comparison to VEGF is used as a specific ligand for Flt-1, similar biological activities in monocytes (here shown as tissue factor production) were observed (Figure 1), which is in concordance with the model of one receptor shared by PlGF and VEGF (Figure 2).

3. IDENTIFICATION OF VEGFR-1 AND VEGFR-2 SPECIFIC ACTIVITIES BY IDENTIFICATION OF VEGF-RECEPTOR SPECIFIC LIGANDS

Shortly after the identification of the VEGFR-1 as a receptor for VEGF, the flk-1/KDR receptor tyrosine kinase was identified as the second VEGF-receptor in endothelial cells (Millauer et al., 1993). In order to assess the biological functions of these receptors for endothelial cells, the VEGFR-1 specific ligand PlGF was compared with VEGF. The maximal activity of VEGF in inducing endothelial tissue factor production is much higher than that observed with PlGF (Figure 1). These data are consistent with the model of Flt-1 as a receptor in monocytes and endothelial cells and Flk-1/KDR as an endothelial cell specific VEGF-receptor (Figure 2). The observation that the PlGF-Flt-1 ligand-receptor complex mediates activity in endothelial cells is not restricted to the induction of procoagulant tissue factor. PlGF also induces proliferation and chemotaxis *in vitro* as well as vascular permeability and angiogenesis *in vivo*, however at significant lower levels (Park et al. 1994; Cao et al. 1995; Sawano et al. 1996; Ziche et al. 1997). In addition, synergistic interaction between VEGF and PlGF have been demonstrated to occur *in vivo* (Carmeliet et al., 2001). Furthermore, the discovery of the Orf-virus encoded protein VEGF-E as a VEGFR-2 specific ligand complemented the tools to distinguish all the activities mediated by these two receptor in endothelial cells (Figure 2). In fact, in endothelial cells VEGF and VEGF-E display comparable activities, whereas PlGF is only a very weak activator of endothelial cells as demonstrated by tissue factor production (Figure 1). Finally, by comparison of VEGF-E with PlGF in vivo biological activities mediated by the endothelial cells can be distinguished from monocyte mediated activities.

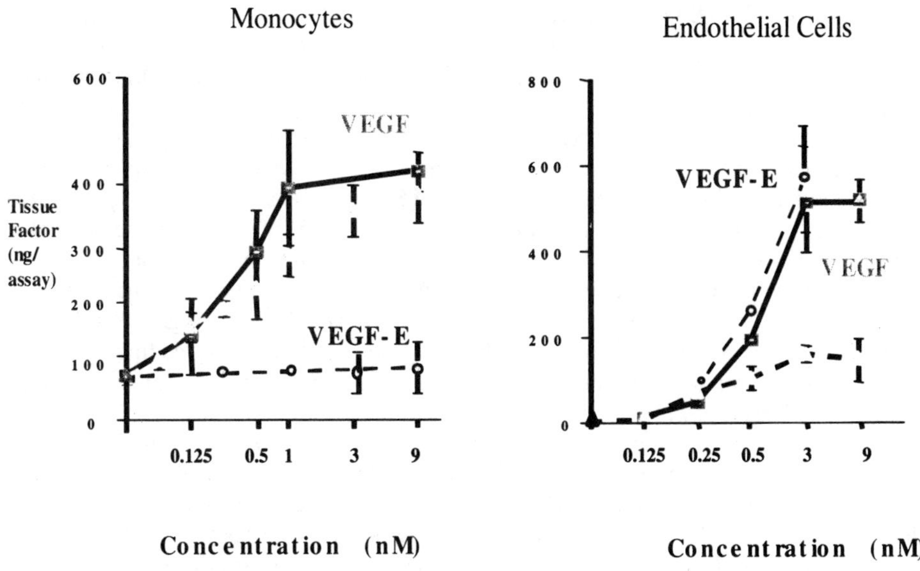

Figure 1. Comparison of PlGF, VEGF and VEGF-E in terms of their ability to activate monocytes and endothelial cells as assessed by tissue factor induction.

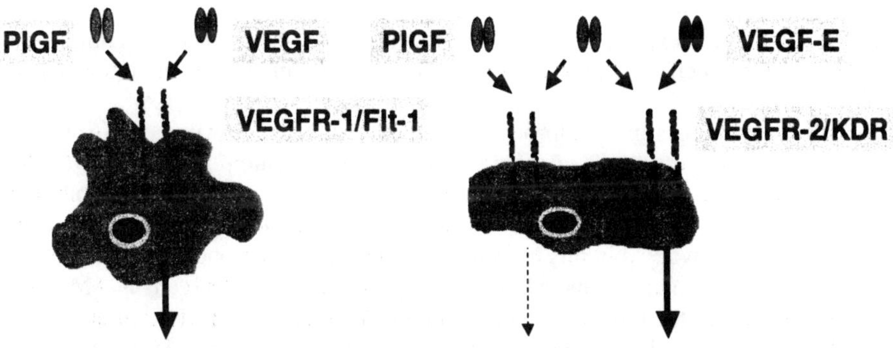

To analyze which VEGF-effects are mediated via monocytes or endothelial cells

Figure 2. Scheme of the VEGFR-1 and VEGFR-2 expression in monocytes and endothelial cells.

4. DISSECTION OF ENDOTHELIAL AND NON ENDOTHELIAL CELL FUNCTIONS BY USE OF VEGFR-SPECIFIC LIGANDS

This principal ability to dissect monocytic from endothelial functions is of relevance to assess the role of non endothelial cells in angiogenesis. For instance both monocytes as well as endothelial precursor cells (EPC) have been implied to contribute to angiogenesis by either enhancing growth or motility of endothelial cells or by direct incorporation into vessels (Asahara et al., 1997; Sunderkotter et al., 1991). In addition to angiogenesis, arteriogenesis was suggested to employ cells different from endothelial cells. Arteriogenesis, the growth of collateral arteries after occlusion of major arteries, is induced after an enormous increase of blood flow and consecutive high shear rates in preexisting arterioles which is caused by the deflected blood pressure gradient. This is believed to start a remodeling process, probably involving monocytes, leading to growth of these vessels. Both surrounding smooth muscle cells as well as endothelial cells have to migrate and proliferate, in order to build a larger vessel which then can work as a natural bypass of the occluded vessel. This process, mimicked in several models, can be enhanced by addition of growth factors. We studied the involvement of monocytes and endothelial cells in the process of VEGF-elicited arteriogenesis. In order to analyze the role of endothelial cells and non-endothelial cells (such as monocytes) by comparing VEGFR-2 with VEGFR-1 selective ligands in the processes of arteriogenesis, we used the chronic ischemic hind limb model in the rabbit. Stimulation with either VEGF or VEGF-E showed increased formation of collateral vessels in comparison to the control. However, stimulation with PlGF turned out to be even more effective than the one observed with VEGF (Figure 3). In fact, the maximal concentrations of PlGF yielded effects not far below the one observed with the strongest arteriogenic factor known so far, which is MCP-1 (Ito et al., 1997). Surprisingly, if PlGF and VEGF-E were combined, no additive effects were observed (Pipp et al., submitt.). These findings indicate that a major contribution for collateral vessel formation results from VEGFR-1 mediated signaling although the VEGFR-2 also appears to participate.

In order to further explore the mechanism underlying these in vivo findings we compared receptor specific ligands in *in vitro* models for monocyte recruitment and angiogenesis.

First, monocyte transmigration through the endothelial cells, grown to confluence on filter membranes, thus creating two compartments, was measured in response to the addition of VEGF and its homologues to the lower chamber. By addition of inhibiting monoclonal antibodies, we identified several adhesion molecules on both endothelium and monocytes being involved in this transmigration process. On monocytes, the integrin receptors LFA-1 (α_L/β_2 integrin) and Mac-1 (α_M/β_2) and on endothelial cells ICAM-1 are the major mediators for the monocyte transmigration. Whereas VEGF (Heil et al., 2000) or PlGF (Pipp et al. submitted) stimulate this transmigration process via an increased expression of these integrins, we could show that treatment with VEGF-E did not affect expression of LFA-1 and Mac-1 on monocytes and did not increase transmigration.

Next, we compared the ability of PlGF to induce angiogenesis *in vitro* by using a sprout formation assay described previously (Nehls and Drenckhahn, 1995). In this assay, all parameters of angiogenesis including proteolytic activation, proliferation, migration and survival of endothelial cells are reflected. In consequence, VEGF is a potent inducer

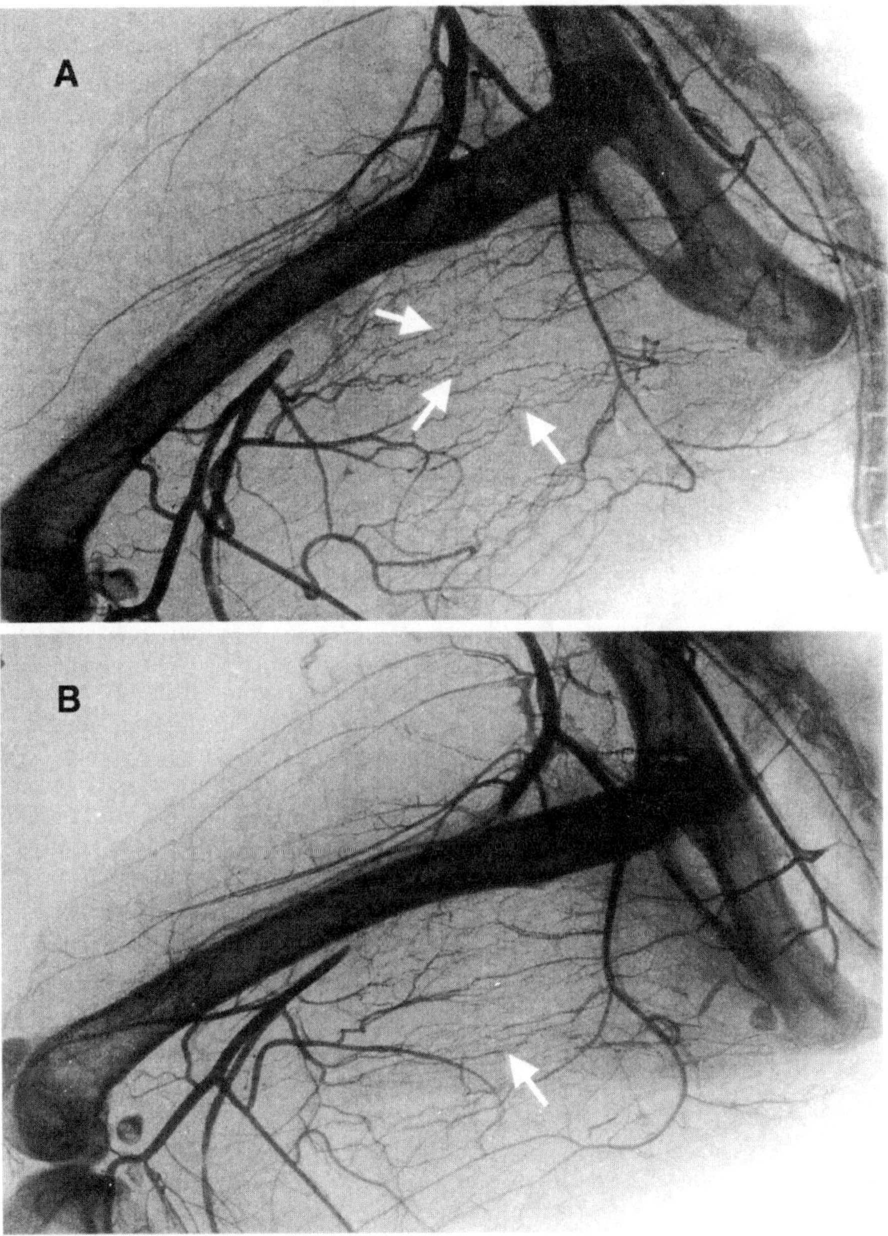

Figure 3. Rabbit angiograms after femoral artery ligation and one week chronic infusion of either A, PlGF (3 µg/kg), or B, VEGF (3 µg/kg), G, VEGF-E (1.5 µg/kg). Whereas with PlGF many collateral vessels are visible (arrows), fewer and smaller can be observed with VEGF.

of sprout formation, a property mediated by the VEGFR-2 because VEGF-E can almost as potent as VEGF induce angiogenesis in this assay. However, the VEGFR-1 specific homologue fails to induce vessel formation in this assay. Interestingly, even combinations of high concentrations of PlGF with VEGF or VEGF-E cannot further enhance the effects of this factor, indicating that the two VEGF-receptors do not cooperate in this system.

5. INVOLVEMENT OF THE VEGF-RECEPTORS VEGFR-1 AND VEGFR-2 IN HEMATOPOETIC STEM CELL MOBILIZATION

The ability of PlGF to induce arteriogenesis even stronger than VEGF and VEGF-E can be explained both by the attraction and activation of monocytes but also by stem cell mobilization. Recently, several publications suggested a contribution of mobilized hematopoietic stem or progenitor cells to processes of blood vessel growth. Asahara and coworkers found that the extent of endothelial progenitor cell (EPC) mobilization and further the neovascularisation can be stimulated by the administration of VEGF (Asahara et al., 1997). These findings can be explained by the effect of VEGF on the proliferation and differentiation of hematopoietic stem cells (Asahara et al., 1999), which is not only giving rise to EPC but also to growth of other blood cell lineages including the monocyte/dendritic cell lineage (Gabrilovich et al., 1998). A recently published report suggests a role of the VEGFR-1 (flt-1) but not the VEGFR-2 (flk1-/KDR) to be responsible for recruitment of hematopoietic stem cells(Hattori et al., 2002). We are currently investigating this issue by using receptor specific VEGF homologues. The information from these experiments may have some clinical relevance. Recently, results from a clinical study were published demonstrating the beneficial effects of Granulocyte Monocyte-Colony Stimulating Factor (GM-CSF) on the growth of collaterals in human hearts. One possible explanation for this observation may be the potency of GM-CSF to stimulate the mobilization of stem cells to the blood, analog to what has been described for VEGF. However, using the ischemic hind limb mouse model for arteriogenesis we were unable to detect any accumulation of bone-marrow derived (stem) cells close to growing collateral arteries (manuscript in preparation).

We could recently demonstrate that reduction of hematopoietic precursor cells lead to strong impairment of arteriogenesis (M. Heil, Am. J. Physiol. in press). This decrease in arteriogenic activity could be rescued by injection of isolated and purified peripheral blood monocytes. Together with the fact that endothelial precursor cells differentiate into endothelial cells in much longer time intervals than used in our study, a functional involvement of monocyte recruitment in arteriogenesis appears to be most likely. Surprisingly, infusion of both VEGF-E as well as PlGF increased the mobilization of hematopoietic precursor cells including EPC and mononuclear cells (manuscript in preparation). This study suggests that infusion of biological substances *in vivo* may have more than one function and disserve careful discussion. Whether PlGF mediated recruitment of EPC contributes to angiogenesis and arteriogenesis needs further investigation (see Figure 4).

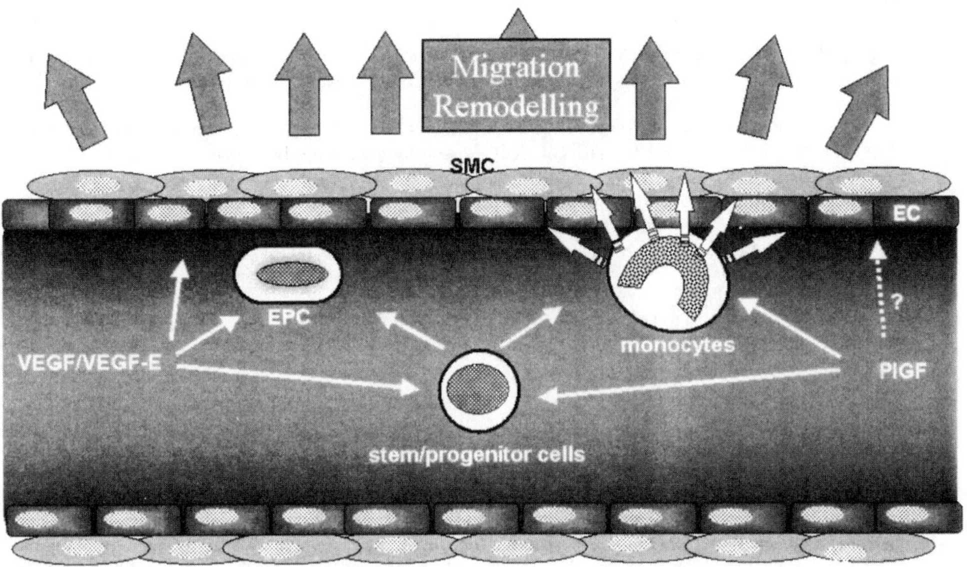

Figure 4. Scheme of the diverse possible involvement of VEGFR-1 and VEGFR-2

6. CONCLUSION

VEGF is the major inducer of angiogenesis with activities on both monocytes and endothelial cells. Based on the hypothesis that the diverse functions of VEGF are related to differential expression and signaling of its two receptors and/or to distinct signaling pathways, we have identified VEGFR-1 and VEGFR-2 selective homologues of VEGF. The VEGF homologue placenta growth factor (PIGF) binds specifically to the VEGFR-1, which is the exclusive VEGF-receptor on monocytes. VEGF-E, a protein encoded by the parapox Orf-virus binds and activates only the VEGFR-2 that is believed to be the major VEGF-signaling receptor in endothelial cells. In consequence, PIGF displays identical activities in monocytes as VEGF, whereas VEGF-E is inactive. In contrast, when human microvascular endothelial cells are tested in an assay for sprouting angiogenesis *in vitro*, VEGF and VEGF-E but not PIGF are angiogenic. In addition, when VEGF-E and PIGF are tested in an animal model for arteriogenesis, PIGF more strongly than VEGF-E can enhance collateral growth. Furthermore, treatment with PIGF induces mobilization of endothelial cells suggesting that the effect of PIGF can in principal be both explained by generation of endothelial cells from precursor cells at sites of arteriogenesis and angiogenesis and by mobilization and differentiation of mononuclear precursor cells to differentiate and function as monocytes. These results suggest that the selective activities of PIGF and VEGF-E can be employed for further identifying the pathophysiological functions of VEGFR-1 or VEGFR-2 expressing hematopoietic progenitor cells.

7. REFERENCES

Asahara, T., Murohara, T., Sullivan, A., Silver, M., van der Zee, R., Li, T., Witzenbichler, B., Schatteman, G., and Issner, J. M., 1997, Isolation of putative progenitor endothelial cells for angiogenesis, Science *275*, 964-967.

Asahara, T., Takahashi, T., Masuda, H., Kalka, C., Chen, D., Iwaguro, H., Inai, Y., Silver, M., and Isner, J. M., 1999, VEGF contributes to postnatal neovascularization by mobilizing bone marrow-derived endothelial progenitor cells, Embo J *18*, 3964-72.

Carmeliet, P., Moons, L., Luttun, A., Vincenti, V., Compernolle, V., De Mol, M., Wu, Y., Bono, F., Devy, L., Beck, H., *et al.*, 2001, Synergism between vascular endothelial growth factor and placental growth factor contributes to angiogenesis and plasma extravasation in pathological conditions, Nat Med *7*, 575-83.

Clauss, M. (1998). Functions of the VEGF receptor-1 (Flt-1) in the vasculature, Trends *Cardiovasc Med 8*, 243-247.

Clauss, M., Gerlach, M., Gerlach, H., Brett, J., Wang, F., Familletti, P. C., Pan, Y.-C., Olander, J. V., Connolly, D. T., and Stern, D., 1990, Vascular permeability factor: A tumor-derived polypeptide that induces endothelial cell and monocyte procoagulant activity, and promotes monocyte migration, JExpMed *172*, 1535-1545.

Clauss, M., and Schaper, W., 2000, Vascular endothelial growth factor: A Jack-of-all-trades or a nonspecific stress gene? [editorial; comment], Circ Res *86*, 251-2.

Gabrilovich, D., Ishida, T., Oyama, T., Ran, S., Kravtsov, V., Nadaf, S., and Carbone, D. P., 1998, Vascular endothelial growth factor inhibits the development of dendritic cells and dramatically affects the differentiation of multiple hematopoietic lineages in vivo, Blood *92*, 4150-66.

Hattori, K., Heissig, B., Wu, Y., Dias, S., Tejada, R., Ferris, B., Hicklin, D. J., Zhu, Z., Bohlen, P., Witte, L., Hendrikx, J., Hackett, N. R., Crystal, R. G, Moore, M. A., Werb, Z., Lyden, D., Rafii, S., 2002, Placental growth factor reconstitutes hematopoiesis by. recruiting VEGFR1(+) stem cells from bone-marrow microenvironment, Nat Med *8*, 841-9.

Heil, M., Clauss, M., Suzuki, K., Buschmann, I. R., Willuweit, A., Fischer, S., and Schaper, W., 2000, Vascular endothelial growth factor (VEGF) stimulates monocyte migration through endothelial monolayers via increased integrin expression, Eur J Cell Biol *79*, 850-7.

Ito, W., Arras, M., Winkler, B., Scholz, D., Schaper, J., and Schaper, W., 1997, Monocyte chemotactic protein-1 increases collateral and peripheral conductance after femoral artery occlusion, Circulation Research *80*, 829-837.

Leung, D. W., Cachianes, G., Kuang, W. J., Goeddel, D. V., and Ferrara, N., 1989, Vascular endothelial growth-factor is a secreted angiogenic mitogen, Science *246*, 1306-1309.

Millauer, B., Wizigmann-Voos, S., Schnürch, H., Martinez, R., Moller, N. P. H., Risau, W., and Ullrich, A., 1993, High affinity VEGF binding and developmental expression suggest flk-1 as a major regulator of vasculogenesis and angiogenesis, Cell *72*, 835-846.

Nehls, V., and Drenckhahn, D., 1995, A novel, microcarrier-based in vitro assay for rapid and reliable quantification of three-dimensional cell migration and angiogenesis, Microvasc Res *50*, 311-22.

Nemerson, Y. (1988). Tissue factor and hemostasis, Blood *71*, 1-8.

Pepper, M. S., Ferrara, N., Orci, L., and Montesano, R., 1991, Vascular endothelial growth-factor (VEGF) induces plasminogen activators and plasminogen-activator inhibitor-1 in microvascular endothelial-cells, BiochemBiophysRe *181*, 902-906.

Risau, W., 1997, Mechanisms of angiogenesis, Nature *386*, 671-674.

Sunderkotter, C., Goebeler, M., Schulzeosthoff, K., Bhardwaj, R., and Sorg, C., 1991, Macrophage-derived angiogenesis factors, PharmTher *51*, 195-216.

CIRCULATING ENDOTHELIAL CELLS AS A NOVEL MARKER OF ANGIOGENESIS

Patrizia Mancuso, Angelica Calleri, Cristina Cassi, Alberto Gobbi, Manuela Capillo, Giancarlo Pruneri, Giovanni Martinelli, and Francesco Bertolini*

1. SUMMARY

Measurement of tumor angiogenesis to predict and/or to assess the efficacy of antiangiogenic therapies is mainly based on the evaluation of microvessel density (MVD). We developed a novel flow cytometry procedure to measure circulating endothelial cells (CECs) and circulating endothelial cells progenitors (CECPs) in either preclinical and clinical studies.

Preclinical studies were performed on an animal model of human lymphoma. A trend toward higher CECs values was observed on day 7 and 14 after transplant, and differences vs controls were highly significant on day 21 (p=0.0061). A strong correlation was found between CECs and tumor volume (r=0.942, p=0.004) and between CECs and tumor-generated VEGF (r=0.669, p=0.02). In mice given cyclophosphamide, most of circulating apoptotic cells were hematopoietic and not endothelial. Conversely, in mice given endostatin, all of the increase in apoptotic cells was in the endothelial cell compartment.

In a parallel study, we looked for CECs in the peripheral blood of 20 healthy controls and 76 newly diagnosed cancer patients by means of four-color flow cytometry. In breast cancer (n=46) and lymphoma (n=30) patients, both resting and activated CECs were increased by 5 fold (P<0.0008 vs control). CECs significantly correlated with plasma levels of VCAM-1 and VEGF. Resting and activated CECs were similar to healthy controls in 7 lymphoma patients achieving complete remission after chemotherapy, and activated CECs were found to decrease in 13 breast cancer patients evaluated before and 24h after quadrantectomy.

In conclusion, our findings indicate a close relation between CEC increase and tumor progression, and support CECs evaluation as a clinically relevant, non invasive angiogenesis marker. Furthermore, this assay offers insight into anti-angiogenic activity of different drugs.

---

* Divisions of Hematology-Oncology, Pathology and Experimental Oncology, European Institute of Oncology, and IFOM-FIRC Institute of Molecular Oncology, Milan, Italy

Novel Angiogenic Mechanisms: Role of Circulating Progenitor Endothelial Cells.
Edited by Nicanor I. Moldovan, Kluwer Academic/Plenum Publishers, 2003.

2. INTRODUCTION

The generation of new blood vessels (angiogenesis) is considered an essential step in tumor growth and metastasis[1], and a new class of drugs with targeted activity on angiogenic vessels has been developed to control cancer progression[2]. At the present time, measurement of tumor angiogenesis to predict and/or assess the efficacy of anti-angiogenic therapies is mainly based on the evaluation of microvessel density (MVD). In this procedure, blood vessels of tumor samples are stained with antibodies and counted by light microscopy. This approach is invasive, MVD of tumor biopsy might not correlate with MVD of the whole tumor specimen, MVD might not be useful to predict the efficacy of an anti-angiogenic drugs[3], and the correlation between MVD and the clinical outcome is still uncertain in most tumor types[4].

In the past, it has been reported that circulating endothelial cells (CECs) are increased in the peripheral blood (PB) of patients affected by sickle cell anemia[5], cytomegalovirus[6] or rickettsial[7] infection, myocardial infarction and endotoxinemia[8, 9]. Moreover, increased CECs have been reported in patients bearing intravascular instrumentation[10].

In our laboratory, we developed a novel flow cytometry procedure to measure CECs and circulating endothelial progenitors (CEPs) in an animal model of human lymphoma and in cancer patients. In parallel, we evaluated CECs viability to ascertain whether this measurement may reflect the antiangiogenic properties of a given drug. Studies were performed in whole blood with commercially available monoclonal antibodies.

3. MATERIALS AND METHODS

3.1. Preclinical Studies

3.1.1. Animal Model

As described previously[11, 12], 6-8 week-old NOD/SCID mice were injected *i.p.* with 10×10^6 Namalwa cells (phenotype CD3-, CD10+, CD13-, CD19+, CD20+, GlyA-). Namalwa cells were derived from an EBV+ Burkitt's lymphoma, obtained from American Type Culture Collection (Manassas, VA) and cultured in RPMI-8% fetal bovine serum (HyClone, Logan, UT). Tumor growth was evaluated every other day, tumors were measured by calipers, and the formula [width^2 x length x 0.52] applied for approximating the volume of a spheroid[12, 13]. To evaluate CECs and circulating human VEGF, Namalwa tumor-bearing NOD/SCID mice and untransplanted controls (n=6 per study group) were bled from the lateral tail vein before and on day 7, 14 and 21 after transplant. All of the procedures involving animals were done in accordance with national and international laws and policies.

3.1.2. Cyclophosphamide (CTX) and Endostatin Treatment

In drug treatment studies, on day 21 after tumor injection drugs were supplied at a site remote from the inoculated tumor. According to previous studies[12], the cytotoxic drug Cyclophosphamide (CTX), (Sigma Chemical Co., St. Louis, MO) was given *i.p.* at the maximum tolerable dose (MTD) of 150 mg/kg as a single administration (n=6), the anti-angiogenic drug endostatin (Calbiochem, san Diego, CA) was given *s.c.* as a single dose of 150 µg/mouse (n=6). As a control, tumor-bearing mice received *i.p.* or *s.c.* PBS (n=6 per study group). Before treatment, and 24h after, mice were bled from the lateral tail vein for CECs evaluation.

3.1.3. Tumor Evaluation

On day 22, mice were sacrificed by CO_2 inhalation. Tumors were collected from all mice and evaluated by histology, immunohistochemistry (IHC) and flow cytometry (FC) as described previously[11, 12]. For histology and IHC evaluation, Namalwa tumor samples were fixed in 10% buffered formalin and embedded in paraffin. Tumor sections (4 µm-thick) were stained with H&E and Giemsa for conventional histology. For IHC, sections were immunostained with anti-CD10 and -CD20 monoclonal antibodies from DAKO (Glostrup, Denmark). Tumor expression of human CD19 and CD20 antigens was also evaluated by FC using BD (Mountain View, CA) monoclonal antibodies. MVD was evaluated as described previously[11]. To detect the area with the highest MVD (hot spot), H&E stained slides were evaluated at x40 and x100. Three microscopic fields were then examined in this area at x250 (each field representing an area of 0.72 mm^2), and the mean MVD value was recorded. Any endothelial cell or endothelial cell cluster that was clearly separated from adjacent microvessels was considered a single, countable microvessel.

3.1.4. Measurement of Murine CECs Number and Viability by FC

Murine CEC were enumerated by three-color FC using a panel of monoclonal antibodies reacting with murine CD45 (to exclude hematopoietic cells) and endothelial murine markers VEGF receptor 2 fetal liver kinase 1 (FLK), CD105, VE cadherin, MECA-32, CD31 and CD34 (PharMingen BD, San Diego, CA). After red cell lysis, cell suspensions were evaluated by a FACSCalibur (BD, San Jose, CA) using analysis gates designed to remove dead cells, platelets and debris. After acquisition of at least 100,000 cells per sample, analyses were considered as informative when adequate numbers of events (i.e., >50, typically 100-200) were collected in the CEC enumeration gates. The percent of stained cells was determined as compared with appropriate negative controls. Positivity was defined as being greater than non-specific background staining. According to the method of Philpott et al.[14], annexin V and 7AAD were used to detect apoptotic and dead cells[11, 12, 14].

3.1.5. Evaluation of Human VEGF in Mouse PB

Human VEGF (known to be produced by Namalwa cells; Ref. 11) was measured in the PB of tumor-bearing mice and controls by commercial ELISA kits (R&D, Minneapolis, MN) as described previously[11].

3.2. Clinical Studies

3.2.1. Patient's characteristics

Peripheral blood was collected in ethylenediaminetetraacetic acid (EDTA) tubes through 21G needles in 76 newly diagnosed cancer patients (30 with lymphoma and 46 with breast cancer, [BC]) and 20 controls. Among lymphoma patients, 28 had B-cell low (n=16, including 8 patients with lymphocytic lymphoma-CLL) or high grade (n=12) non-Hodgkin's lymphoma, 2 had Hodgkin's disease. Five lymphoma patients (1 mantle cell, 1 marginal zone, 3 lymphocytic lymphoma-CLL) had leukemic disease. Among 46 BC patients, all with infiltrating duct carcinoma, 9 were N0, 10 had axillary lymph node metastases, 27 had distant metastatic diseases. Patients bearing intravascular instrumentation were excluded from the study.

3.2.2. Measurement of human CEC number by FC

A panel of human monoclonal antibodies including anti-CD45 to exclude hematopoietic cells, anti-CD31, -CD34, -CD36, -CD105, -CD106, -CD133, -P1H12[5, 17], and appropriate analysis gates (Fig. 1) were used to enumerate resting and activated CECs and CEPs. Monoclonal antibodies (Tab. 1) were conjugated with FITC, R-Phycoerythrin (PE), PerCP or allophycocyanin (APC), and cell suspensions evaluated by a FACSCalibur equipped with a second red-diode laser (BD, San Jose, CA). Absolute cell numbers were calculated by reference fluorescent beads and "lyse-no-wash" procedures used to increase sensitivity and reproducibility[18]. After acquisition of at least 100,000 cells per PB sample, analyses were considered as informative when adequate numbers of events (ie >100, typically 3-400) were collected in the CECs enumeration gates.

3.2.3. Definition of Resting and Activated CECs

Resting CECs were defined as negative for hematopoietic marker CD45; positive for endothelial markers P1H12, CD31 and CD34; negative for activation markers CD105 and CD106 and negative for the progenitor marker CD133. Activated CECs were defined as CD45-, P1H12+, CD31+, CD34+, CD105 or CD106+, CD133-. According to Rafii[19], CEPs were depicted by expression of CD133. Although some of the monoclonal antibodies used in our CEC panel (namely CD31, CD34, CD105 and CD133) react with defined hematopoietic cell populations in addition to CECs, the P1H12 monoclonal antibody is highly specific as an endothelial marker. Unlike other commonly used endothelial markers, P1H12 specifically localizes to endothelial cells of all vessels including cancerous tissues and does not react with hematopoietic or epithelial cells[17]. Regarding activated CEC markers, high levels of CD105 (endoglin), a receptor for transforming growth factor beta, and vascular cell adhesion molecule-1 (VCAM-1) are currently considered as hallmarks of activated endothelial cells either in vitro and in tissues undergoing angiogenesis in vivo[20-21].

3.2.4. Sensitivity and Specificity of our Procedure

Sensitivity and specificity of our procedure were evaluated by serial dilution of human umbilical cord endothelial cells (expressing an "activated CEC" phenotype) in the U-937 cell line. The detection limit of our procedure was 0.1 cell/µL, and specificity was>90%. Anti-CD34 antibodies conjugated with APC, when compared with PE, have decreased mean fluorescence intensity[18]. Although the large majority of CD34+

hematopoietic progenitors were excluded from our analysis gate by CD45 expression[18], APC-conjugated anti-CD34 was useful to discriminate between the very tiny population of CD45- haematopoietic progenitors, which were CD34$^{+++(bright)}$, and CD34^{+} CECs (Fig.1).

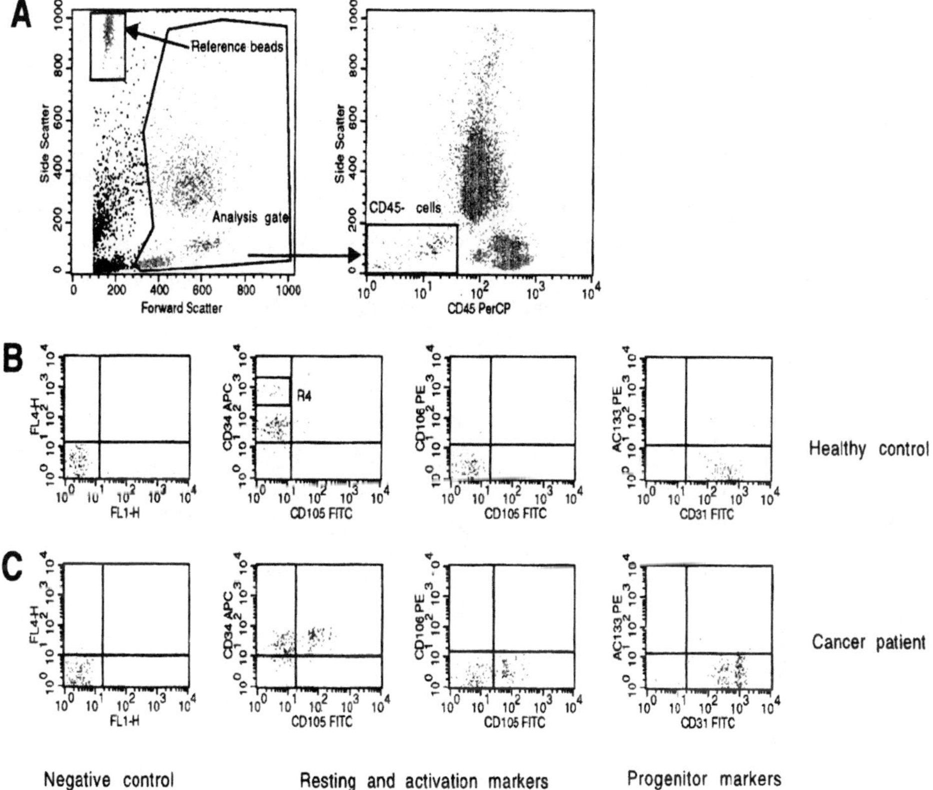

Fig. 1: Four-color flow cytometry evaluation of circulating endothelial cells and endothelial progenitors (from ref. 35, modified). Representative top panel on the left shows the analysis gate used to exclude platelets, death cells and debris and the reference beads used to obtain absolute cell count. Top panel on the right shows the gate used to exclude hematopoietic cells expressing the CD45 antigen. Middle and bottom panels indicate negative controls and the expression of antigens used to evaluate resting (CD31 and CD34), activated (CD105 and CD106) and progenitor (CD133) endothelial cells. Middle panels show the resting phenotype of a representative healthy control, bottom panels show the more activated phenotype of a representative newly diagnosed breast cancer patient. R4 indicates CD45- haematopoietic progenitors depicted by high CD34 expression.

Table 1: Target antigens, related cluster designations, antibody clones and conjugation of human monoclonal antibodies used in the study.

Antigen	Cluster designation	Antibody clone	Conjugation
PECAM-1[1]	CD31	WM59 (Pharmingen BD)	FITC
gp 105-120	CD34	HPCA-2 (BD)	APC
LCA[2]	CD45	2D1 (BD)	PerCP
Endoglin	CD105	8E11 (Euroclone)	FITC
VCAM-1[3]	CD106	5110C9 (Pharmingen BD)	PE
AC133	CD133	AC133/1 (Miltenyi)	PE
P1H12	Not yet designated	P1H12 (Chemicon)	FITC

3.2.5. Evaluation of MVD

Microvessel density was evaluated by anti-CD34 staining in paraffin-embedded tumor samples as we described in detail elsewhere[22]. In brief, sections were immunostained with CD34-reactive Qbend/10 (Signet Laboratories, Dedham, MA). The substitution of the primary antibody with non immune mouse serum was used as negative control. For MVD enumeration, at least 10 fields were evaluated at x250 (0.78 mm^3). Any brown-staining endothelial cell (or cluster) that was clearly separated from adjacent microvessels was considered a single, countable microvessel and vessel lumens were not a prerequisite to define a structure as a microvessel. In duplicate independent readings, MVD intrareader variability was found to be 14±10% (r=0.879).

3.2.6. Evaluation of human VEGF and VCAM-1

Circulating VEGF and VCAM-1 were measured in the plasma of patients and controls by commercial ELISA kits (R&D, Minneapolis, MN, and BioSource, Camarillo, CA, respectively) as we previously described[23]. It has been suggested in the past that VEGF measurements in EDTA-plasma samples may in part reflect VEGF release from activated platelets. As described by Wynendaele et al[24], however, EDTA may influence platelet shape, but no statistically significant difference in VEGF levels is observed in plasma samples collected with EDTA *vs.* plasma samples collected with four different anticoagulants (sodium citrate, theophylin, adenosine, dipyridamole) to obtain maximal platelet stabilization.

3.3. Statistical Analysis

CEC kinetics were compared in tumor-bearing mice and untransplanted controls over the entire period of observation. Statistical comparisons were performed using the *t* test, ANOVA and linear regression when data were normally distributed and the non-parametric analyses of Spearman and Mann-Whitney when data were not normally distributed. Values of P lower than 0.05 were considered to be statistically significant.

4. RESULTS

4.1. CECs Kinetics in Controls and Xenografted Mice

In the CD45 negative fraction of non-hematopoietic cells, expression of CD31, CD34, VE-cadherin and MECA-32 was similar to FLK expression. Thus, throughout the

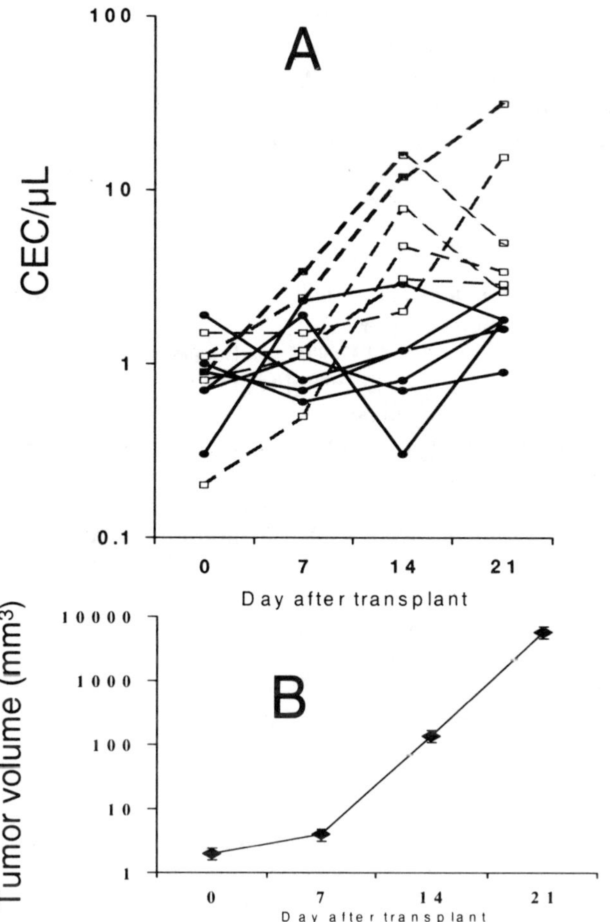

Figure 2 A: CEC kinetics in NOD/SCID mice injected with Namalwa lymphoma cells (n=6) and in controls (n=6) progenitors (from ref. 34, modified). Despite repeated bleeding, CEC were stable in untransplanted control mice (solid lines). In tumor-bearing animals (dotted lines), a trend toward increased CEC numbers was already observed on day 7 and 14 after transplant, and on day 21 differences were highly significant (p=0.0061 vs control).
B: Namalwa tumor growth curve. Values are reported as mean ±1SD.

study CECs are reported as CD45- FLK+ cells. Before transplant, mean CECs/µL were 0.9 (95% confidence limit 0.6-1.1). As indicated in Fig.2, a trend toward higher CECs values was observed in xenografted mice on day 7 and 14, and differences were highly significant on day 21, when in xenografted mice mean CECs/µL were 10.2 (95% confidence limit 1.2-19.3, p=0.0061 vs controls). A strong correlation was found between CECs and tumor volume (r=0.942, p=0.004 by Spearman Rank test) and between CEC and tumor weight on day 21 (r=0.885, p=0.01). In control mice, circulating human VEGF was undetectable, in tumor-bearing mice mean human VEGF was 14 pg/mL (95% confidence limit 6-22). A positive correlation was found in tumor-bearing mice between CECs and human VEGF (r=0.669, p=0.02) and between MVD and tumor volume (r=0.948, p=0.05). The correlation between CECs and MVD was slightly weaker (r=0.737, p=0.26). Between 30-60% of CECs expressed the activation marker CD105, and differences between tumor-bearing mice and controls were not significant.

4.2. Murine CEC Viability

As shown in Fig. 3, in control mice most CECs were annexin V+, and 30-50% of them also expressed intermediate 7AAD staining. These findings suggest that in healthy mice most CECs may have initiated an apoptotic process. In tumor-bearing mice, the mean frequency of annexin V+ or 7AAD+ CEC was 29% (95% confidence limit 23-35%, p<0.01 vs control). This finding indicates improved CEC viability in tumor-bearing mice, possibly because of high VEGF levels generated by tumor cells.

As indicated in Fig. 4, the administration of the cytotoxic drug CTX at MTD (n=6 CTX-treated mice and 6 tumor-bearing, untreated mice evaluated as control) was associated 24 h after treatment with a significant increase of circulating cells showing intermediate and high levels of 7AAD staining. After CTX administration at MTD, ~ 85% of the 7AAD+ apoptotic cells were hematopoietic and not endothelial (CD45+ FLK-), and ~ 40% of FLK+ CECs were still viable (7AAD-). Conversely, 24 hours after the administration of the anti-angiogenic drug endostatin (n=6 endostatin-treated mice and 6 tumor-bearing, untreated mice evaluated as control), all of the increase in 7AAD+ circulating cells was in the endothelial (CD45- FLK+) cell compartment, and most of the CECs were apoptotic or dead, i.e., expressing high 7AAD staining (p<0.001 vs controls).

4.3. Human CECs Determination

In healthy controls (n=20), mean values of resting and activated CECs were 7.9/µL (95% confidence interval [CI] 4.7-11.1), and 1.2/µL (95% CI 0.1-2.3), respectively. Seven female controls were reevaluated during the menstrual period associated with physiological active angiogenesis. Mean activated CECs were found to increase from 2.4/µL (95% CI, <0.1-5.5) to 4.4/µL (95% CI<0.1-10.5). However, this trend did not reach statistical significance (*P*=0.15 by Wilcoxon matched pairs test).

In 76 newly diagnosed patients, mean resting and activated CECs were 39.1/µL (95% CI 16.8-61.4) and 6.8/µL (95% CI 5.0-8.6), ie increased by 5 fold (*P*<0.0008 vs control by ANOVA). CEC distribution was normal in controls and skewed in patients. Three of 5 lymphoma patients in leukemic phase contributed to most of the skewing observed in CEC distribution among patients; lymphoma patients, compared to BC patients, had higher mean resting (78.0/µL, [95% CI 22.8-133.5] vs 15.8/µL [95% CI

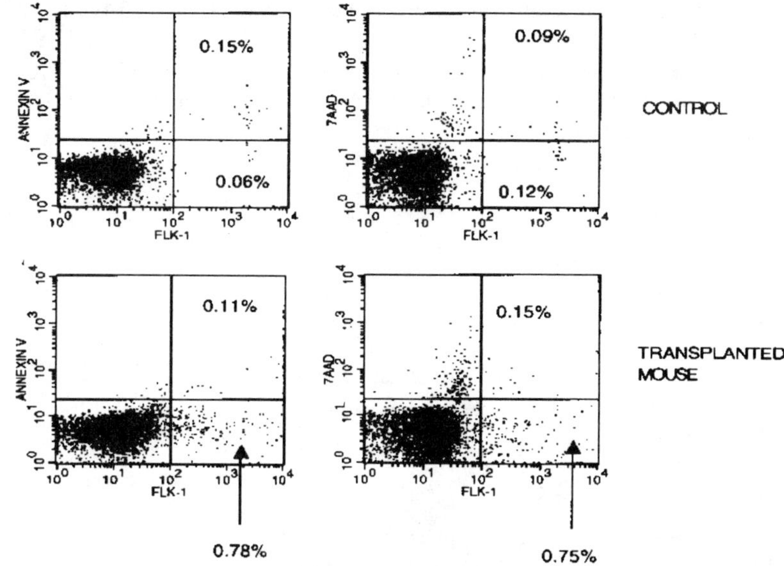

Fig. 3: Representative evaluation of CEC viability in control NOD/SCID mice (top panels) and in mice bearing Namalwa lymphoma (bottom panels, progenitors (from ref. 34, modified)). In control mice, the majority of CEC were annexin V positive, and 30-50% of them also expressed intermediate 7AAD staining. Accordingly, in control mice most CEC may have initiated an apoptotic process. In tumor-bearing mice, the frequency of annexin V and 7AAD indicated that most CEC were viable

12.0-19.7], P=0.0078 by ANOVA) and activated (8.7/µL, [95% CI 5.1-12.3] vs 5.6/µL, [95% CI 3.7-7.4], P=0.18) CECs.

Differences between BC patients with early or metastatic diseases were not significant. In controls and patients the number of CECs did not significantly increased with age. Studies are ongoing to fully understand the clinical features associated with the particularly elevated CEC values observed in some patients, and repeated CEC measurements in patients and controls indicated a low longitudinal CEC variation. Evaluation of CD36 expression showed that in patients and controls at least half CEC were microvascular in origin[5]. In patients and controls the count of resting and activated CEC did not correlate with the count of white cells, red cells or platelets.

4.4. Correlation between VEGF, MVD and CECs

VEGF is produced by most tumor cells[15-16] and is involved in CEP mobilization[25]. Mean VEGF was 83 pg/mL (95% CI, 27-140) and 192 (95% CI, 103-281) pg/mL in controls and patients, respectively (P=0.03 by ANOVA). Correlation between MVD and VEGF and between MVD and CECs did not reach statistical significance. On the other hand, a positive correlation (r=0.419, P=0.009 by multiple regression) was found between CECs per microliter and plasma VEGF. As shown in Fig. 5, a normal distribution of resting CECs, activated CECs and plasma VEGF was observed in controls, whereas a switch to increased VEGF, increased CECs and activated CEC phenotype was observed in cancer patients. Circulating VCAM-1, a glycoprotein produced by angiogenic endothelial cells, was significantly increased in patients (mean 1496 ng/mL, [95% CI, 1161-1831]), compared with controls (838 ng/mL, [95% CI 737-938], P=0.003). VCAM-1 strongly correlated with CECs per microliter (r=0.582, p<0.0001) but not with MVD, and lymphoma patients had significantly higher VCAM-1 levels compared with those with BC (p=0.002).

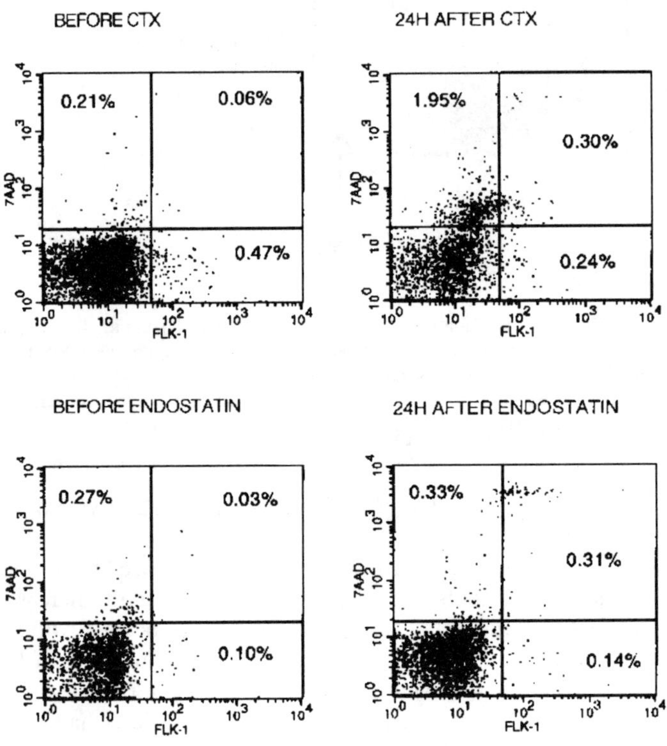

Fig.4: Representative evaluation of CEC viability before (left) and after (right) administration of the cytotoxic drug CTX (top) and of the anti-angiogenic drug endostatin (bottom, from ref. 34, modified). In mice given CTX at MTD, most of the circulating apoptotic (7AAD+) cells were hematopoietic (FLK-) and not endothelial (FLK+), and a relevant frequency of CEC were still viable (FLK+ 7AAD-). In mice given endostatin, all of the increase in circulating apoptotic cells was in the endothelial (FLK+) cell compartment, and most FLK+ CEC were apoptotic (intermediate 7AAD staining) or dead (high 7AAD staining).

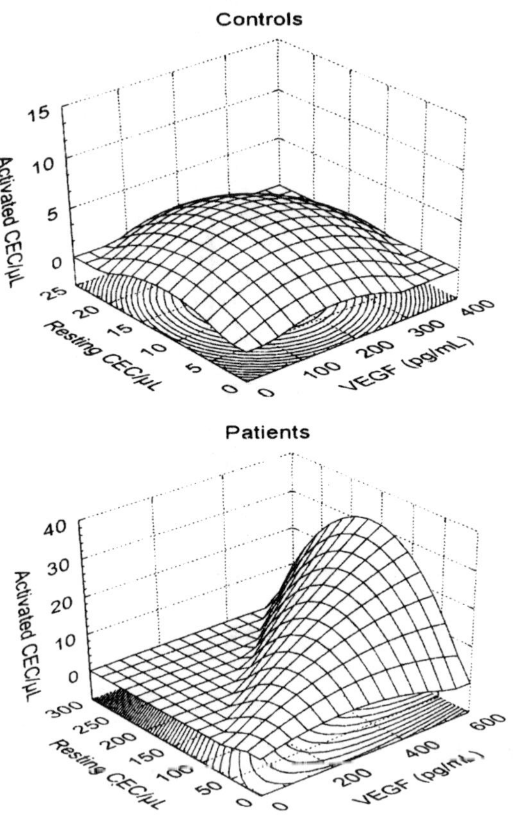

Fig. 5: Three-dimension surface plots showing plasma VEGF, resting and activated circulating endothelial cells (CEC) in healthy subjects and cancer patients (from ref. 35, modified). A normal distribution was prevalent in controls, whereas a switch to increased VEGF, increased CEC and an activated CEC phenotype was observed in cancer patients.

CECs were found to be similar to control values in 7 lymphoma patients who achieved complete remission after chemotherapy. In these patients, mean resting and activated CEC/µL were 12.8/µL (95% CI, 4.0-21.6) and 0.8/µL (95% CI, 0.4-1.2), respectively (P=0.0001 and 0.63 vs newly diagnosed patients and healthy controls, respectively). Furthermore, CECs were found to decrease in 13 BC patients evaluated before and 24 hours after quadrantectomy (Fig. 6). In these BC patients, activated CECs significantly decreased from 9.0/µL (95% CI, 2.4-15.5) to 2.0/µL (95% CI 0.9-3.1, P

=0.0107 by Wilcoxon matched pairs test), whereas mean resting CECs decreased from 25.3/µL (95% CI, 16.3-34.4) to 16.4/µL (95% CI, 10.0-22.8), and statistical significance was borderline (*P*=0.0546).

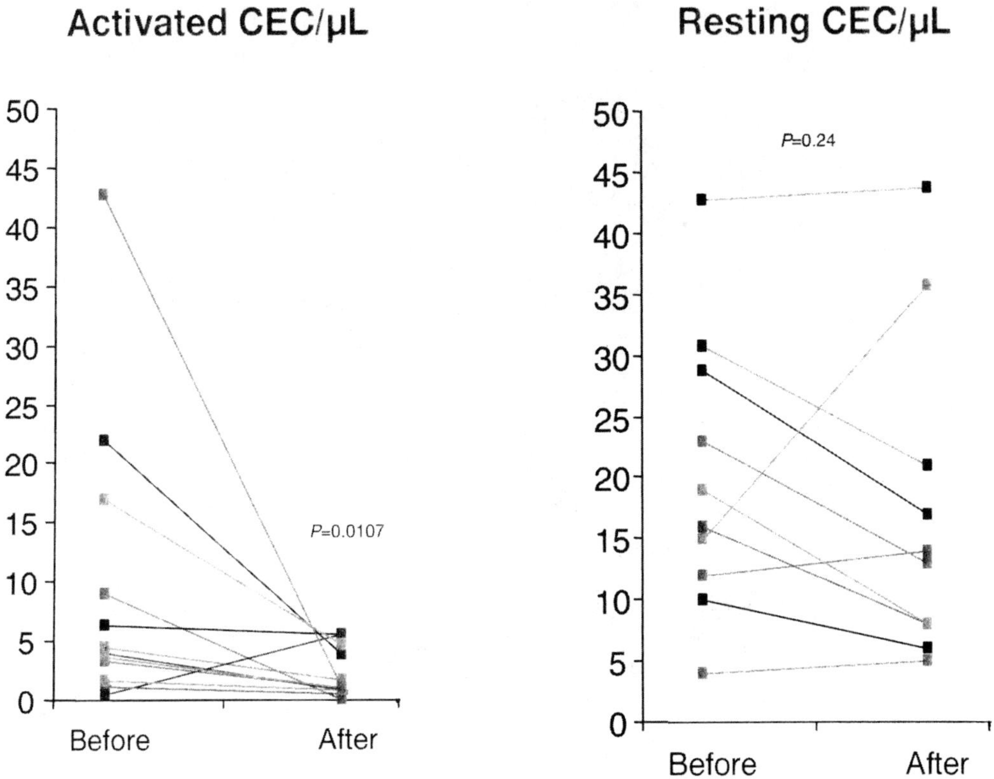

Fig. 6: Circulating endothelial cells (CEC) in 13 breast cancer patients before and after quadrantectomy (from ref. 35, modified). A decrease was observed in both activated and resting CEC. *P* was calculated by the Wilcoxon matched pairs test.

Regarding CEPs, they were <0.5/µL in all controls and newly diagnosed patients evaluated. Higher CEP counts were found in 4 out of 11 patients evaluated while recovering from high-dose chemotherapy-induced aplasia and in 2 out of 7 healthy controls evaluated during the menstrual period. In these 6 cases, CEP values ranged from 1.1 to 9/µL.

5. DISCUSSION

Despite its importance as a prognostic indicator in untreated tumors, MVD has not been shown to be a valid measure to guide or evaluate antiangiogenic treatment. We took advantage of an animal model of human lymphoma[11, 12] to evaluate CEC kinetics and viability before and after drug therapy. Present data indicate a stable CEC increase after lymphoma transplant, and the strong correlation observed between CEC and tumor volume indicates that CEC increase may parallel tumor progression. As shown in Fig. 2, some variability in CEC numbers was found among different tumor-bearing_mice. The correlation observed between CEC and circulating levels of human VEGF (produced by transplanted Namalwa cells, ref. 11), suggests that this variable may also play a role in determining CEC frequency in tumor-bearing mice. The role of VEGF is particularly interesting, because we have found that in control animals most CECs seem to have initiated an apoptotic program, whereas CEC viability is markedly improved in tumor-bearing mice. Considering the antiapoptotic properties of VEGF[26], this growth factor might play a relevant role in preserving CECs from apoptosis.

In a previous work, the frequency of endothelial apoptotic cells (measured by anti-FLK monoclonal antibodies, 7AAD staining, and FC) was found to be significantly increased in Namalwa tumors removed from NOD/SCID mice treated with the anti-angiogenic drug endostatin[12]. In the present work we evaluated CEC viability before and after drug therapy, and found that the cytotoxic drug CTX at MTD induces apoptosis of circulating hematopoietic and (to a lesser extent) endothelial cells. Conversely, the anti-angiogenic drug endostatin specifically targets endothelial and not hematopoietic cells. Thus, the measurement of CEC viability during clinical studies might be of relevant help to define the balance between cytotoxic and anti-angiogenic activity of different drug schedules.

Regarding results obtained in cancer patients, Increased CECs have been described so far only in conditions that have in common the presence of vascular injury[5, 10]. Our finding that resting and activated CECs are increased in newly diagnosed cancer patients and decline after cure underlines the crucial role of angiogenesis in both solid tumors and hematopoietic malignancies. Moreover, resting and activated CECs appear to be novel and promising surrogate angiogenesis markers. Interestingly, our data about the increase of activated (CD105 or CD106+) CECs in cancer patients offer a rationale for recent reports about the predictive potential of soluble CD105 and CD106 in the PB of BC patients[28, 29].

CEC increase in cancer patients may be due to at least three different reasons: CEC may derive from the lining of angiogenic tumor vessels, represent ingress of proliferating endothelial cells from neighboring normal tissue or derive from distant uninvolved vessels activated by tumor's derived cytokines. Chang et al.[27] have recently provided evidence indicating that tumor blood vessels may be mosaics in which both endothelial and tumor cells form the luminal surface. Although controversies still exist about the frequency of tumor cells contributing to this phenomenon[30], data by Chang et al[27] provide a possible explanation for the finding of high CEC numbers in cancer patients. In their colon tumor xenograft model, in fact, they collected morphological evidence of endothelial cell shedding from the lining of tumor vessels. Commenting data on mosaic tumor vessels, Folkman[31] has indicated that in tumor angiogenic vessels the endothelial cell lining is continuously migrating, whereas in mature, quiescent vessels there is little or no endothelial cell turnover. Again, this picture fits well with our present data on CEC kinetics.

Taken together, our findings support CEC evaluation as a surrogate, non invasive angiogenesis marker that may contribute to the existing panel of angiogenesis assays[32]. The measurement of CEC viability by FC seems a useful, non-invasive tool to evaluate the efficacy of targeted anti-angiogenic drugs in preclinical models of human disease as well as in clinical trials. Considering that CEC correlate well with tumor volume and circulating VEGF, known to be a relevant prognostic factor in human lymphoma[23,33], we are evaluating CEC longitudinally in patients enrolled in different clinical trials. The measurement of CEC viability is currently under investigation to ascertain whether a given drug therapy has antiangiogenic properties or not.

6. ACKNOWLEDGMENTS

Supported by AIRC and FIRC.

7. REFERENCES

1. J. Folkman, Angiogenesis in cancer, vascular, rheumatoid and other diseases,*Nat. Med.* **1**:27-31, 1995.
2. J. Folkman, P. Hahnfeldt, and J. Hlatky, Cancer: looking outside the genome, *Nat. Rev. Mol Cell Biol.* **1**: 76-79, 2000.
3. L. Hlatky, P. Hahnfeldt and J. Folkman, Clinical Application of Antiangiogenic Therapy: Microvessel Density, What it does and doesn't tell us, *J Natl Cancer Inst.* **94**:883-893, 2002.
4. N. Weidner, Angiogenesis as a predictor of clinical outcome in cancer patients, *Hum. Pathol.* **31**:403-405, 2000.
5. A. Solovey, Y. Lin, P. Browne, S. Choong, E. Wayner and Hebbel RP, Circulating endothelial cells in sickle cell anemia, *New Engl J Med.* **337**:1584-1590, 1997.
6. A. Grefte, M. Van der Giessen and W. van Son, The TH. Circulating cytomegalovirus-infected endothelial cells in patients with an active CMV infection, *J Infect Dis.* **167**:70-277, 1993.
7. M. Drancourt, F. George, P. Brouqui, J. Sampol and D. Raoult, Diagnosis of Mediterranean spotted fever by indirect immunofluorescence of Rickettsia conorii in circulating endothelial cells isolated with monoclonal antibody-coated immunomagnetic beads, *J Infect Dis.* **166**:660-663, 1992.
8. M. Mutin, I. Canavy, A. Blann, M. Bory, J. Sampol and F. Dignat-George, Direct evidence of endothelial injury in acute myocardial infarction and unstable angina by demonstration of circulating endothelial cells, *Blood.* **93**:2951-2958, 1999.
9. Y. Lin, D.J. Weisdorf, A. Solovey and R.P. Hebbel, Origins of circulating endothelial cells and endothelial outgrowth from blood, *J Clin Invest.* **105**:71-77, 2000.
10. F. George, P. Poncelet, J.C. Laurent, O. Massot, D. Arnoux, N. Lequeux, P. Ambrosi, C. Chicheportiche and J. Sampol, Cytofluorometric detection of human endothelial cells in whole blood using S-Endo 1 monoclonal antibody, *J Immunol Methods.* **139**:65-75, 1991.
11. L. Fusetti, A. Gobbi, C. Rabascio, G. Pruneri, N. Carboni, F. Peccatori, G. Martinelli and F. Bertolini, Human Myeloid and Lymphoid Malignancies in the Non-Obese Diabetic/Severe Combined Immunodeficiency Mouse Model: Frequency of Apoptotic Cells in Solid Tumors and Efficiency and Speed of Engraftment Correlate with Vascular Endothelial Growth Factor Production, *Cancer Res.* **60**:2527-2534, 2000.
12. F. Bertolini, L. Fusetti, P. Mancuso, A. Gobbi, C. Corsini, P.F. Ferrucci, G. Martinelli and G.Pruneri, Endostatin, an antiangiogenic drug, induces tumor stabilization after chemotherapy or anti-CD20 therapy in a NOD/SCID mouse model of human high-grade non-Hodgkin's lymphoma, *Blood.* **96**:282-287, 2000.
13. T. Bohem, J. Folkman, T. Browder and M.S. O'Reilly, Antiangiogenic therapy of experimental cancer does not induce acquired drug resistance, *Nature.* **390**:404-407, 1997.
14. N.J. Philpott, A.J.C. Turner, J. Scopes, M. Westby, J.C.W. Marsch, E.C. Gordon-Smith, A. G. Dalgleish and F.M. Gibson, The use of 7-amino actinomycin D in identifying apoptosis: Semplicity of use and broad spectrum of application compared with other techniques, *Blood.* **87**:2244-2251, 1996.
15. J. Folkman,. Incipient angiogenesis, *J Natl Cancer Inst.* **92**:94-95, 2000.
16. D. Hanahan and R.A. Weinberg, The hallmarks of cancer, *Cell.* **100**:57-70, 2000.

17. B. St Croix, C. Rago, V. Velculescu, G. Traverso, K.E. Romans, E. Montgomery, A. Lal, G.J. Riggins, C. Lengauer, B. Vogelstein and K.W. Kinzler,. Genes expressed in human tumor endothelium, *Science*. **289**:1197-1202. 2000.

18. O. Fornas, J. Garcia and J. Petriz, Flow cytometry counting of CD34+ cells in whole blood, *Nat Med*. **6**:833-836, 2000.

19. S. Rafii, Circulating endothelial precursors: mystery, reality, and promise, *J Clin Invest*. **105**:17-19, 2000.

20. C. Li, I.N. Hampson, L. Hampson, P. Kumar, C. Bernabeu and S. Kumar, CD105 antagonizes the inhibitory signaling of transforming growth factor beta1 on human vascular endothelial cells, *FASEB J*. **14**:55-64, 2000.

21. L. Osborn, C. Hession, R. R. Tizard, C. Vassallo, S. Luhowskyj, G. chi-Rosso and R. Lobb, Direct expression cloning of vascular cell adhesion molecule 1, a cytokine-induced endothelial protein that binds to lymphocytes, *Cell* **59**:1203-1211, 1989.

22. G. Pruneri, F. Bertolini, D. Soligo, N. Carboni, A. Cortelezzi, P.F. Ferrucci, R. Buffa, G. Lambertenghi-Delilers and F. Pezzella et al. Angiogenesis in myelodysplastic syndromes, *Br J Cance*. **81**:1398-1401, 1999.

23. F. Bertolini, M. Paolucci, F. Peccatori, S. Cinieri, A. Agazzi, P.F. Ferrucci, E. Cocorocchio, A. Goldirsch and G. Martinelli, Angiogenic growth factors and endostatin in non-Hodgkin's lymphoma, *Br J Haematol*; **106**:504-509, 1999.

24. W. Wynendaele, R. Derua, M.F. Hoylaerts, A. Pawinski, E. Waelkens, E.A. Bruijn, R. Paridaens, W. Merlevede and A.T. van Oosterom, Vascular endothelial growth factor measured in platelet poor plasma allows optimal separation between cancer patients and volunteers: A key to study an angiogenic marker *in vivo?*, *Ann Oncol* **10**: 965-971, 1999.

25. T. Asahara, T. Takahashi, H. Masuda, C. Kalka, D. Chen, H. Iwaguro, Y. Inai, M. Silver and J.M. Isner, VEGF contributes to postnatal neovascularization by mobilizing bone marrow-derived endothelial progenitor cells., *EMBO J*. **18**:3964-72, 1999.

26. N. Ferrara, and T. Davis-Smyth, The biology of vascular endothelial growth factor., *Endocrine Rev*, **18**: 4-25, 1997.

27. Y.S. Chang, E. di Tomaso, D.M. McDonald, R. Jones, R.K. Jain, and L.L. Munn, Mosaic blood vessels in tumors: frequency of cancer cells in contact with flowing blood, *Proc. Natl. Acad. Sci. USA*. **97**: 14608-14613, 2000.

28. C. Li, B. Guo, P.B. Wilson, A. Stewart, G. Byrne, N. Bundred and S. Kumar, Plasma levels of soluble CD105 correlate with metastasis in patients with breast cancer, *Int J Cancer* .**89**:122-6, 2000.

29. G.J. Byrne, A. Ghellal, J. Iddon, A.D. Blann, V. venizelos, S. Kumar, A. Howell and N.J. Bundred, Serum soluble vascular cell adhesion molecule-1: role as a surrogate marker of angiogenesis, *J Natl Cancer Inst*. **92**:1329 36, 2000.

30. D.M. McDonald and A.J.E. Foss, Endothelial cells of tumor vessels: Abnormal but not absent, *Cancer and metastasis reviews* **19**: 109-120, 2000.

31. J. Folkman, Can mosaic tumor vessels facilitate molecular diagnosis of cancer?, *Proc. Natl. Acad. Sci. USA*, **98**: 398-400, 2001.

32. R. Auerbach, N. Akhtar, R.L. Lewis and B. L. Shinners, Angiogenesis assays: problems and pitfalls, *Cancer and metastasis reviews*, **19**: 167-172, 2000.

33. P. Salven, A. Orpana, L. Teerenhovi. And H. Joensuu, Simultaneous elevation in the serum concentrations of the angiogenic growth factors VEGF and bFGF is an independent predictor of poor prognosis in non-Hodgkin lymphoma: a single-institution study of 200 patients, *Blood*. **96**:3712-3718, 2000.

34. S. Monestiroli, P. Mancuso, A. Burlini, G. Pruneri, C. Dell'Agnola, A. Gobbi, G. Martinelli and F. Bertolini, Kinetics and viability of circulating endothelial cells as surrogate angiogenesis marker in an animal model of human lymphoma, *Cancer Res*. **61**:4341-4, 2001.

35. P. Mancuso, A. Burlini, G. Pruneri, A. Goldhirsch, G. Martinelli and F. Bertolini, Resting and activated endothelial cells are increased in the peripheral blood of cancer patients, *Blood*. **97**:3658-3661, 2001.

TISSULAR INSEMINATION OF PROGENITOR ENDOTHELIAL CELLS: THE PROBLEM, AND A SUGGESTED SOLUTION

Nicanor I. Moldovan*

1. SUMMARY

The contribution of circulating precursor endothelial cells (CPEC) to adult angiogenesis is now well established. However, the mechanism of their tissular engrafting remains poorly understood. The classical paradigm of "sprouting" cannot accommodate the main features of the CPEC-based angiogenic process. Additionally, vasculogenesis based on the differentiation of angioblasts, as defined in the embryonic stages, is not applicable to adult neo-vascularization either. In search for a solution to this dilemma, I suggest that the ability of monocytes/macrophages to produce tunnels, as effect of their protease-dependent migration in the extracellular matrices, is instrumental for the tissular insemination of CPEC. Here I present in vivo and in vitro experimental evidence for the existence of tunnels, and for their colonization by monocytes/macrophages and by other cells, including CPEC. As a paradigm of CPEC behavior, the tunneling model (in an extended sense) may also explain the propagation of the endothelium with arteriolar phenotype within the pre-existent downstream capillary network. Thus, the sprouting mechanism might be a valid explanation for the formation of new capillaries and venules, whereas CPEC would contribute mostly, if not exclusively, to the extension of arteriolar branches of microvasculature. Adult angiogenesis occurs therefore as a multifunctional process based on intercellular cooperation, in which there are involved endothelial cells (EC) or their precursors, as well as other cell types. In specific circumstances, the lumen (i.e. the tunnel) may occur before the "definitive" microvessel. Therefore the very notion of microvessel may need to be extended, to include the tunnels.

---

*Davis Heart and Lung Research Institute, The Ohio State University, Columbus, OH, 43210

Novel Angiogenic Mechanisms: Role of Circulating Progenitor Endothelial Cells.
Edited by Nicanor I. Moldovan, Kluwer Academic/Plenum Publishers, 2003.

2. BACKGROUND

CPEC contribute to maintenance and remodeling of microvasculature in the adult animals[1-6]. One piece of still missing knowledge regarding the involvement of CPEC in the formation of microvasculature, besides their true nature and origin, is the mechanism of their tissular engraftment, or insemination.

The textbook model of angiogenesis is sprouting[7]. In this model, a single cell type (endothelial) is able to fulfill all the functions needed to produce a new capillary branch. Sprouting is conceived to begin, as effect of specific angiogenic growth factors, with the dissolution of the endothelial basement membrane by the cells themselves, and to continue with the outward sending of a cytoplasmic projection. The mobilization of EC, expressed in the disruption of confluency, is expected to trigger cellular proliferation[8]. Formation and fusion of intracellular vacuoles would explain the occurrence of the lumen of new microvessels[9]. In principle, a newly-formed branch was supposed to be functional right after its occurrence, but the details of this stage of angiogenesis are scarce.

In real life situations, the contribution of endothelial proliferation (overall important, and in which so much research effort has been put), seems to be dispensable for the very early steps of angiogenesis. Microvascular extensions can occur without EC proliferation, at least in some models, for a good period of time before the establishment of a fully developed microvessel[10]. Cellular motility and redistribution, with penetration of the matrix by migrating cells, are more significant for those early stages of angiogenesis[11].

Depending on the tissular location where the sprouting takes place, the sequence of events, and even the cellular partners involved may vary. For example, in post-capillary venules, the first step in sprouting is the dismantling of the pericytes layer[12]. Importantly, the process takes place in the presence and with contribution of macrophages, which were shown to create a space between pericytes and endothelium. These macrophages migrate later in the interstitium[12].

In other models, the pericytes were regularly found at, and in front of, the advancing tips of endothelial sprouts. Their processes were suggested to serve as guiding structures, aiding the outgrowth of EC[13, 14]. In a study done on the budding molars of 2-day old rats, pericyte-like cells were constantly found in "caves" where the capillaries were located, or destined to be located[14].

It is important to note that the pericytes themselves are a vaguely defined cell population, being related either to smooth muscle cells, to fibroblasts, or to macrophages, Pericytes seem to derive from macrophages the brain[15], and they are related to the osteoblasts of the bone[16].

The picture became even more complicated when it was realized that other cells, specifically the mononuclear CPEC, contribute to the formation of the angiogenic tufts. This contribution presents a number of features that have to be accounted for. The most important is the circulatory (hematopoietic/monocytic) nature, i. e. CPEC are thought to derive mostly from the bone marrow[17]. CPEC as new cellular additions may be initially non-proliferative, as discussed before[10]. Related to the circulatory nature of CPEC, it could be the mosaic pattern of their engraftment[18, 19]. This means a spotty attachment, as opposed to a continuous coverage of the microvessel, which would be expected from the clonal expansion of a sprout. Another important feature is that when CPEC suspensions are injected in the tissues, during cell therapy protocols, they end up in the walls of functional microvessels, or in angiogenic tufts. This suggests that CPEC may engraft in the new microvessels also from the outside, not only from the blood front[3]. Paradoxically, intra-tissular injection of pure suspensions of mature, differentiated EC apparently fails to incorporate them in pre-formed microvessels, or to induce neovascularization[20]. Intercellular cooperation might be again needed.

Also important is the realization of the existence of a cooperation between EC and monocytes or macrophages[21]. In this context it should be noted the detection at the tips of microvessels of metalloelastase (matrix metalloprotease 12, or MMP12), which is a monocyte/macrophage specific enzyme[22]. Thus, the macrophages may help the penetration of sprouts into dense tissues. This is a key function necessary for capillary extension, and fulfilled either by EC themselves, or by pericytes. It was clearly described even in angiogenesis models based on pure EC cultures[23].

Composite models of angiogenesis were advanced, where a sprouting-like process, starting from a parent vessel, was conceived as incorporating the contribution of CPEC[24]. However, the rationale for such a heterogeneous mechanism was never provided. The closest similar situation is that of "maintenance angiogenesis", addressing the replacement of damaged EC in larger vessels[5] (see also Gunsilius, Chapter 3 of this volume). Nevertheless, while perfectly suited to explain the turn-over and repairing of the endothelial lining, the applicability of this model to sprouting angiogenesis is debatable. There is no obvious reason for which the new sprouts or microvascular tufts formed from actively proliferating EC, would already need bone-marrow "replacements" and/or additions.

The possibility remains that the rate of EC proliferation even in the most actively growing capillaries is too low to fulfill urgent needs for new blood supply, and therefore more "building blocks" or "helpers" are recruited from the blood, or from the nearby microvessels.

Alternatively, we propose the tunneling mechanism[25,26] as a solution to the problem of tissue engraftment of CPEC. The emphasis is put on the role of mononuclear cells of monocyte/macrophage phenotype, and specifically on their ability to create behind them, during migration, lasting "empty" (or of lower density) spaces. The tunnels can be formed either by migratory cells during tissue penetration, or by other mechanisms (for example as leftovers of former capillaries, which have lost their cellular walls). The second tenet of this model is that the tunnels could be subsequently populated by other blood-derived cells, including CPEC, or even by fresh, more mature EC. The factors controlling monocyte migration and the dissolution of extracellular matrix, as well as those inducing cell arrest, adhesion and spreading (such as the chemoattractants MCP-1, VEGF or others), would also control the tunneling activity, and its angiogenic consequences. Tunneling may take place in the extracellular space such as the extracellular matrix of a tissue, the "provisional matrix" of a tumor[27] or in clots, during their reorganization and resorbtion.

This paper will focus on the factual evidence for tunneling: existence of tunnels, their colonization by cells, and presumed functionality. Then, we will suggest two applications of the tunneling model, one in the recanalization of clots, and another in the extension of arterioles.

3. THE TUNNELING MODEL

We derived the earliest indication for tunneling from the analysis of monocyte recruitment in the hypercholesterolemic rabbit intima, in an ex vivo model of diapedesis. We noted instances where below the attached monocytes the endothelium, the basement membrane and the internal elastic membrane were very thin, suggestive for a powerful proteolytic activity of these cells in the process of penetration   (L. Moldovan and N. Moldovan, 1986, unpublished data).

A more recent confirmation of the notion that tissular migration of mononuclear phagocytes may produce spaces of lower density in the extracellular matrix, i. e., tunnels, came from the observations on experimentally transplanted hearts. In a project on the cellular mechanisms of transplant vasculopathy, we found that Fas-mediated apoptosis of medial smooth muscle cells of microvessels of donor tissue, is involved in the early stages of this pathological process[28]. One of the consequences of the immune infiltration, as seen in histological sections, was sometimes a system of empty spaces within the media of arterioles, and around them. A likely explanation, supported by in vitro data, was that infiltrating monocytes/macrophages would induce the Fas-mediated apoptosis of medial smooth muscle cells (Moldovan et al., 1997, unpublished observations), and then

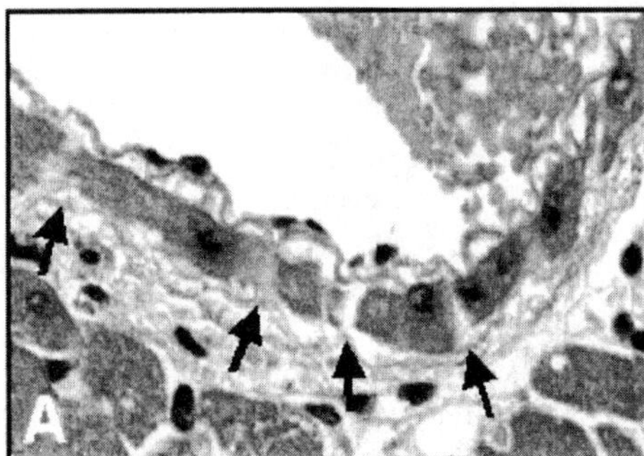
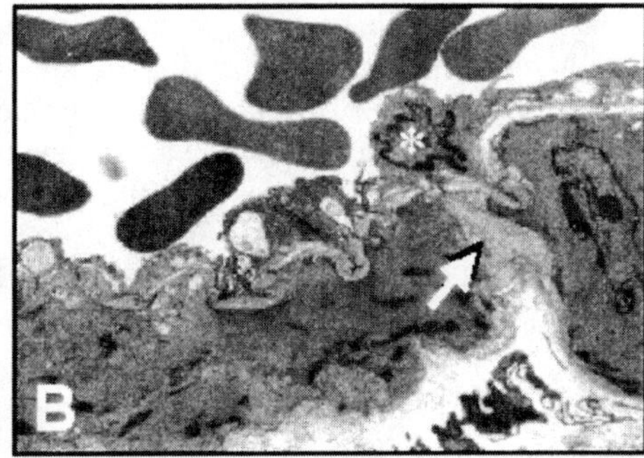

Figure 1. Discontinuities in the organization of smooth muscle cells layers in microvessels of MCP-1 mice, suggestive for recurrent pathways (tunnels) used by monocytes in their diapedesis and perivascular accumulation. A. Histological section; the arrows indicate breaks in medial layer (Elastic van Gieson staining). B. Electron micrograph displaying a mononuclear cell (star) at the entrance of a tunnel (arrow). Original magnifications: A, x120; B, x700.

remove their debris by phagocytosis, leaving behind well defined spaces of lower density (tunnels).

The tunneling concept was further consolidated during the analysis of transgenic mice expressing MCP-1 under the cardiac-specific myosin heavy chain promoter[25, 29]. Particularly intriguing in this mouse model of inflammatory heart failure were the apparent discontinuities of medial smooth muscle cells in some microvessels (Fig. 1 A). Associated with these "breaks" in smooth muscle cell layers, we have often found mononuclear cells (Fig. 1B).

This observation reinforced the previous one, regarding the potentially lasting effect of monocytes/macrophages migration, and of their phagocytosis of other cells, on the tissue structure. Moreover, when we followed the tracks of deeper penetration of these cells within the cardiac tissue, we found evidence for significant but spatially confined tissue degradation, with separation of myocytes, and creation of an intercellular space. This space of reduced density, appeared to be readily filled by cellular debris, or by other intact cells displaying a migratory phenotype (data not shown).

Further immunocytochemical analysis indicated that the tunnel-forming cells are most likely macrophages that secrete the potent, wide-spectrum metalloelastase (MMP12). We found MMP12 positive cells residing in the tubular "empty" spaces of the tunnels, and caught in transversal or longitudinal sections[25].

4. TUNNELS IN ORGANIZED ATRIAL THROMBI

The notion of tunneling offers a fresh perspective to the interpretation of some features present in histological sections of organizing clots, or of granulation tissue. We addressed the organization of atrial thrombi, either in a model of heart failure in the spontaneous hypertensive rat (SHHF)[30], or in the previously described mouse model of inflammatory heart failure[29]. In both instances, in the final stages of the disease there is both formation and organization of intra-atrial thrombi. In these old clots we detected proteolytic rims surrounding the inflammatory cells, but not the myofibroblasts. The myofibroblasts seemed to be firmly attached to the extracellular matrix of granulation tissue, while the proteolytic rims around the inflammatory cells were suggestive for tunneling (Moldovan et al., in preparation).

Another important finding was the presence of erythrocytes in endothelium-free spaces within organized rat atrial clots, while some other erythrocytes were confined within normally endothelium lined capillaries. The analysis of atrial clots in MCP-1 mice revealed similar findings, i. e. the presence of tunnels apparently created by monocytes, and also erythrocytes associated with them.

The common supposition is that the newly formed capillaries are so fragile that they may become "leaky" for erythrocytes. Instead we interpret this observation based on the tunneling mechanism, considering the ability of migrating monocytes/macrophages to facilitate the passive squeezing of the fluid and erythrocytes within the tunnels created by them. Other in vivo and in vitro experiments support this possibility (Moldovan et al, in preparation).

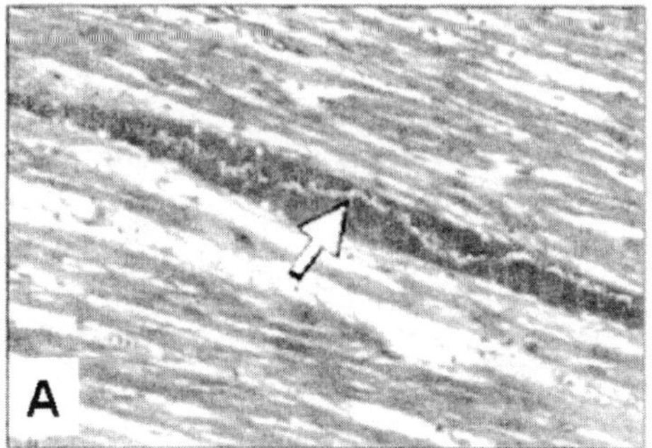

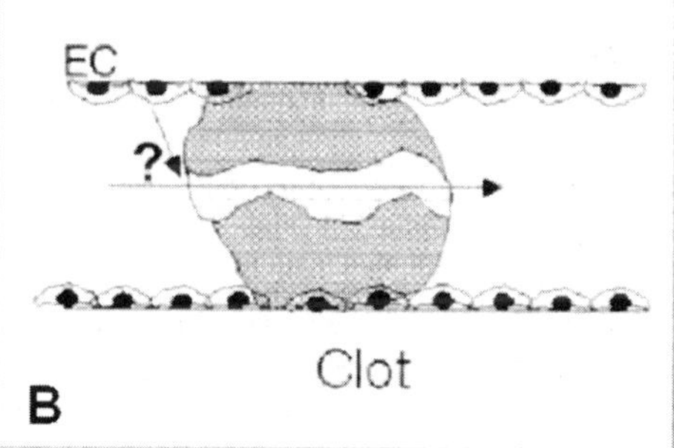

Figure 2. Tunneling in organizing thrombi. A. Longitudinal section through a tunnel filled with leukocytes and erythrocytes in a fibrin clot developed within a coronary branch in a human patient suffering of ischemic heart disease. B. Cartoon describing the topographical constraint imposed on the blood conduits of recanalized clots, and the unlikeness that their endothelium to derive *by sprouting* from the parent vessel. A. Hematoxylin-eosin staining. Original magnification, x120.

The model of monocyte-drilled, leukocyte and erythrocyte-filled tunnels, suggests a mechanism of formation of secondary vessels in the process of reperfusion or recanalization of old clots. This is an important, but so far unexplained observation in vascular pathology. Most often the veins (and sometimes also the arteries) occluded by clots, become recanalized by one or more blood conduits running inside and parallel with the parent vessel (for example, in the Kawasaki syndrome[31]). These secondary vessels are patent and functional, potentially saving the patient's organs, or life. Nevertheless, from a topological point of view it is difficult to understand how they are formed, just because the blood flows in parallel with the original vessel. It is hard to believe that they are derived by sprouting from the EC of parent vessel, because the lumen of such a microvessel would face outward from the parental one (Fig. 2B). Instead, they may be produced by blood cells having consistent proteolytic activity, such as the monocytes/macrophages, and able to penetrate the clot from one side to another. These cells would create tunnels, which thereafter would become enlarged and colonized by other blood elements, possibly including CPEC. An indication on how this may happen, is derived from observations on sections through the myocardium of a patient who suffered from ischemic heart disease (Fig. 2A). An obstructed microvessel displaying an extended intravascular coagulation crosses this micrograph. The clot is permeated longitudinally by a column of mononuclear cells, occasionally incorporating erythrocytes as well. They all reside within an endothelium-free tunnel with the diameter of about a cell's size (20 μm). The original endothelium is still detectable on the margins of the clot.

The tunneling mechanism would also explain the ability of monocytes to penetrate deep in non-vascularized tissues beyond 200 μm, which is hypoxia limit. If erythrocytes can follow the monocytes in tunnels, this cooperation will function as a sort of "emergency" microcirculation, providing the monocytes with a minimum of oxygen supply.

In the experiments where Fas-deficient hearts from mice of the *lpr* phenotype[32] were transplanted in wild-type recipients, we found that the media of arterial microvessels was much better preserved, the infiltration was reduced, and the tunnels did not appear[28]. Instead, another important observation was made. While Fas-positive cells were expected to occur only in the blood perfusing the transplanted organ, in fact they were also sporadically present in an endothelial position, covering the luminal side of blood vessels of the graft. Since the Fas gene cannot be expressed in the *lpr* tissues[32], the only remaining explanation is that circulating cells from the wild type recipient mouse contributed to the re-endothelialization of the (injured?) intima of the transplanted heart. This finding is in agreement with the notion of "fallout endothelialization", described for artificial[33] and natural [34] vascular grafts, and with that of "maintenance angiogenesis"[5].

In addition, we collected evidence from the mouse MCP-1 hearts[25], and from the SHHF rat model of heart failure[30], that the tissular fields displaying tunnels also present signs of neovascularization, apparently with the contribution of bone marrow derived cells. For example, we assessed the distribution of cells expressing the Thy-1 antigen, considered a marker for both hematopoietic cells[35], and for neo-vascularization when present in the endothelium[36]. We found this marker on mononuclear cells in interstitial and luminal positions, as well as in intermediate ones (Fig. 3C, D). This observation supports the possibility that blood-derived CPEC may travel into tissues as part of the inflammatory infiltrate, and end up by edging the lumens of microvessels or of tunnels, attaching from the outside. This would explain the ability of injected CPEC to incorporate in neovascular foci, as mentioned before. A less likely alternative is that "activated" EC would detach and penetrate individually the extracellular matrix.

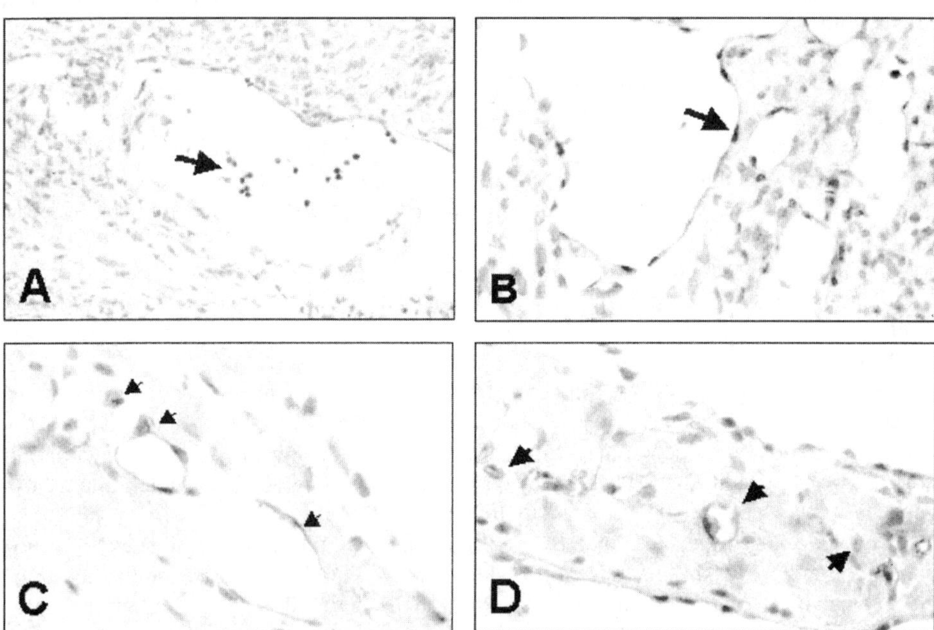

Figure 3. Contribution of CPEC to neo-vascularization in adult animals. A, B. Recipient blood-derived mononuclear cells engrafting in the intimal layer of a transplanted mouse heart. The images represent immunostaining for the Fas marker (black), present only in the cells of the recipient animal. A. Fas-positive leukocytes (arrow) are aggregated in a clot in the lumen of a microvessel from the Fas-deficient (lpr) transplanted heart. Note that in this section the endothelium of the transplanted vessel is negative for Fas. B. Another section in the same lpr transplant, shows Fas-positive cells in an endothelial position (arrow) and Fas-positive infiltrating mononuclear cells. C, D. Expression of the hematopoietic marker Thy-1 (arrowheads, black) in neo-angiogenic fields in failing MCP-1 hearts (C) and in SHHF rats (D). In C, the distribution of positive cells relative to the lumen of a microvessel (outside, tangential. luminal) suggests a stepwise incorporation from the outside. A-D, hematoxylin counterstaining (in gray). Original magnifications, x120. For a color representation of this figure, see color insert at the end of book.

5. TUNNELING IN MATRIGEL

We obtained evidence regarding the various instances of tunnels formation by migrating mononuclear cells, from experiments where we implanted subcutaneously in mice plastic chambers filled with Matrigel (modified after Dvorak et al.[37]). We found in the gel cells migrated through the porous wall of the chamber. These cells produced a moth eaten pattern of empty spaces (tunnels), confined behind the inflammatory front. The tunnels were torturous structures, and they were found cut in different aspects either longitudinally, obliquely, or transversely, a morphological requirement to differentiate them from simple tissular folds[38]. They usually contained cells, but sometimes they looked empty, most likely because of the localization of the sectioning plane through this complex three-dimensional structure. The deepest advanced cells, apparently creating and occupying the tunnels, were mostly mononuclear cells which often retained a monocyte morphology (kidney-like nucleus). Smaller mononuclear and polymorphonuclear cells were also found within the chambers, but their proportion is relatively small (Moldovan *et al.*, in preparation).

We also found erythrocytes entering the chambers, without evidence of capillary formation. Most of the erythrocytes were aligned within the tunnels in straight cords. Apparently, they could squeeze through the chamber's porous wall, accumulate in the space underneath and probably passively follow the fluid filling the tunnels during the penetration of inflammatory cells, as discussed before.

The tunneling process could be reproduced in vitro, using Matrigel and THP-1 monocytes. We incubated THP-1 cells on top of Matrigel for a week or more. Then we fixed and sectioned the gel, and analyzed it microscopically. We found a pattern of cell columns penetrating the gel, one cell following another, accompanied in this case by proliferation (since THP-1 is a proliferative cell line). The process of penetration was amplified by the presence of MCP-1 in the gel.

We also devised a lateral viewing of the in vitro tunneling process. This was obtained by making small wells in the Matrigel layer, then filling them with THP-1 cells which were allowed to penetrate the gel. Cell columns developed during the incubation time, showing that the cells prefer to migrate in the gel one after another. Supposedly, they follow the "leader" cell, i. e. the one making the tunnel.

Since we found the same pattern in various in vivo and in vitro instances, this supports the hypothesis that the cells could take advantage, probably based on a simple biomechanical mechanism, of an easier penetration if they follow one another in a preformed tunnel. Moreover, when we put anti-coagulated human blood, diluted with tissue culture medium, on top of Matrigel pre-penetrated by the THP-1 cells for several days, we saw columns of erythrocytes also penetrating the Matrigel. Hemoglobin-free cells were found at the leading edge of the erythrocyte rouleaux, arguing that the penetrating monocytes can be passively followed by erythrocytes in the tunnels, as suggested by the in vivo data (Moldovan et al., in preparation).

6. DISTRIBUTION OF CPEC IN INFLAMMATORY INFILTRATES

In order to obtain details on the contribution of CPEC to angiogenesis, and on the potential involvement of tunneling mechanism, we took advantage of the transgenic mice expressing beta-galactosidase (B-gal), or the green fluorescent protein (GFP), under the EC-specific Tie2 promoter[39]. From the blood of GFP-Tie2 mice stimulated with VEGF[40] we isolated a mononuclear cell fraction by Hystopaque centrifugation. Among these cells, a subgroup which were larger and more readily to adhere on glass (a feature of monocytes), were also more fluorescent, suggesting the presence of an active Tie2 promoter in this monocyte subpopulation (Fig. 4A). A similar cell suspension isolated from non-stimulated Tie2 B-gal mice was further cultivated on collagen. Among these cells, some became positive for B-gal (Tie2) within 10 days (Fig. 4B). Combined, these data support the expression of the Tie2 endothelial marker in circulating bone marrow derived mononuclear cells of Tie2 B-gal mice.

In these mice we also injected Matrigel subcutaneously, to induce an angiogenic response[41]. As expected, we found Tie2 positive blood vessels penetrating the gels at their periphery, and also identified a strong perivascular inflammation. Among the cells composing this infiltrate, we found Tie2 positive cells with a well preserved monocyte morphology Those cells were different from the more mature macrophages (based on the staining for F4/80 antigen, a macrophages marker[42]), therefore they are probably CPEC (data not shown)..

Deeper in Matrigel, we found cords of mononuclear cells aligned one after another. They were not associated with capillaries, and we could not detect capillaries in those regions. This pattern was reminiscent of the disposition of monocytes in tunnels in vitro.

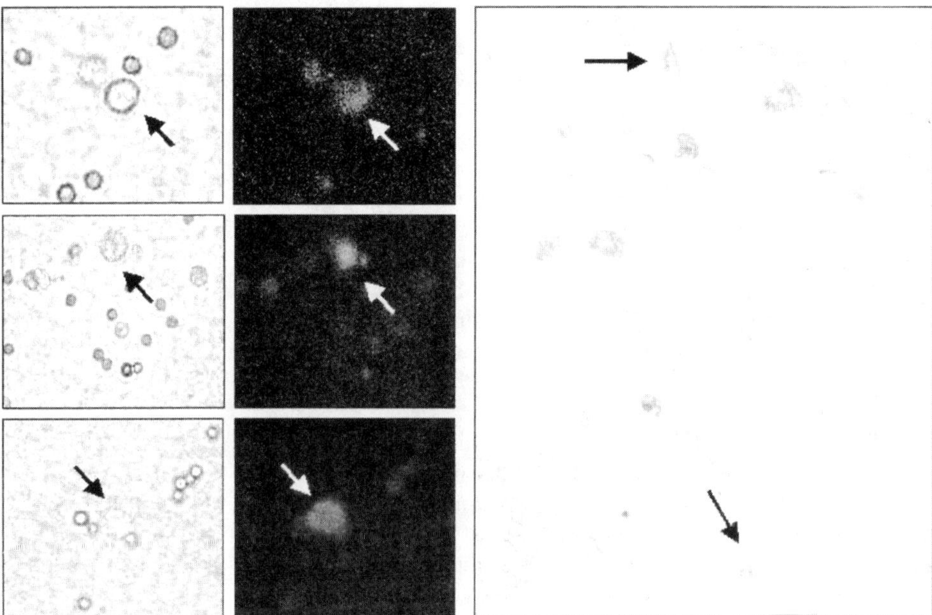

Figure 4. Expression of Tie2 in peripheral blood mononuclear cells. A. Positive cells detected in the fresh isolate from a Tie2-GFP mouse as large, adherent mononuclear cells (arrows). Left column, phase contrast; right column, fluorescence microscopy. B. Presence of an active Tie2 promoter in adherent mononuclear cells cultured for 10 days from the blood of a Tie2 B-gal mouse. The dark color is the substrate of B-gal. Some cells tend to acquire an elongated, spindle cell like morphology (arrows). Original magnifications, x80.

The staining for the macrophage marker F4/80 revealed formation of tunnels lined by macrophages. These structures also displayed sporadic presence of Tie2 positive cells, possible precursors for further development of microvessels as angiogenic tufts.

7. ANGIOGENESIS MODELS IN THE TIE2 B-GAL MOUSE

When studying the architecture of the new microvascular structures, particularly with reference to the validity of the sprouting model, an integral view of the microscopic field of interest becomes essential. In this instance, tissue sectioning may be inappropriate.

Moreover, the analysis of the microvascular endings only from the blood side (as done by perfusions, and by polymeric casts) may be misleading. This is because these techniques will miss the angiogenic events taking place before the connection of a given cellular structure, or branch, to the main perfused conduit. In these circumstances, a two-dimensional model of angiogenesis using pre-labeled cells would be ideal. We selected as such an experimental model the mesentery of Tie2 B-gal mice.

In this setting, the tunneling model was also found potentially relevant for angiogenesis, during the formation and/or preservation of the identity of arteriolar endothelium. Here it does not refer to the penetration of the extracellular matrix and to creation of a lumen, but to its second tenet, i. e. the colonization of a pre-formed lumen by CPEC.

It is known that a microvascular lumen, either before of after it acquires an established endothelial covering, may be re-occupied by other EC. These situations occur, for example, during the advancement of a capillary front in a fibrin gel by a "tug-of-war" type of movement called "guided migration"[43], or when diabetic capillary ghosts are re-colonized by retinal EC[44].

It is known that arterial EC have a different molecular composition versus venular ones. An example is the distribution of ephrinB2 and its receptor EphB4, expressed on the arteriolar and on venular endothelium, respectively[45]. Equally important is the fact that arteriolar capillaries are not neutral, but they belong to either one of the two categories. They may stain halfway for marker, or contain isolated cells expressing ephrins[45]. The question is what does create and maintain the identity of each cell in a given capillary? It is hard to conceive that diffusible factors are the sole explanation, because they would influence more uniformly the cells within a capillary. Therefore, one should consider the origin of cells, besides their location.

We analyzed the expression of Tie2 within the vascular tree of the mesenteric fat of Tie2 B-gal transgenic mice, and we found it unevenly distributed. We observed that the fat tissue, known as an actively angiogenic milieu[46], contains many round, isolated individual B-gal positive cells, which potentially are CPEC[19]. Alternatively, spindle-shaped cells occurred in the process of forming connections among these cells and with the upstream continuous arteriolar endothelium. We believe that this is an example of how CPEC attach within a pre-existent lumen, most alike the way it would happen within a tunnel (Anghelina et al., in preparation).

Emigration of leukocytes takes place at the level of post-capillary venules in designated organs. When they stop in capillaries, they may produce leukostasis[47]. Nevertheless, if the leukocytes (including CPEC) are fewer, they would not produce an obstruction of the blood flow except for a short period of time, until they adhere to the lumen of the capillary. This may happen either on top of an existing endothelium or in between EC, pushing them apart. Alternatively, CPEC may simply squeeze along with the blood, and if the signals for recruitment are not strong enough, they will depart from microvascular beds through the venous compartment, for another round of the circulatory loop.

What controls these processes of recruitment and incorporation of CPEC in an angiogenic bed, is not known at this time. However it is conceivable that there are specific signals, either soluble or on the cell surface, involved in this mechanism, and acting more efficiently in angiogenic tissues than in others. These signals may also act as differentiation factors, therefore during the time spent within microcirculation, CPEC may begin their endothelial maturation, even if they are still circulating cells (see also Schatteman and Awad, Chapter 2; and Mancuso et al.,Chapter 9 of this volume).

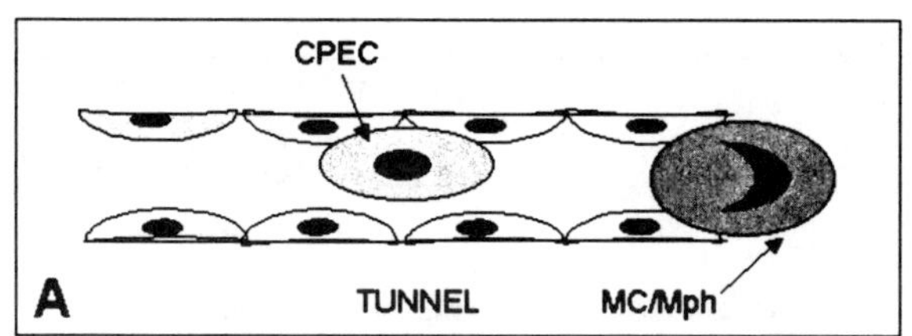

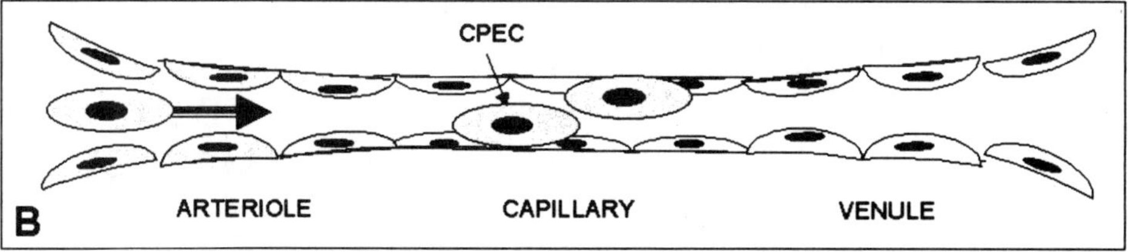

Figure 5. Hypothetical similarity in the behavior of CPEC during the incorporation in both tunnels and in capillaries. A. Tunnel produced by a monocyte/macrophage in a dense extracellular matrix and covered by incidental cells (white). Among them may be CPEC (dark) which may attach, acquire an elongated morphology, and proliferate. B. Capillary populated by CPEC carrying an arterial phenotype (derived either from the bone marrow, or dislodged from the upstream endothelium). These CPEC would adhere to the EC of the capillary and displace some of them. The common theme between A and B is the pre-existence of a lumen which can accommodate the newly coming CPEC. Not to scale.

Otherwise, CPEC derived either from the bone marrow or from the upstream arterial endothelium, would colonize the capillaries of angiogenic tissues, flatten and extend backwards cytoplasmic projections until they reach the nearby arteriolar endothelium. By this mechanism, the arteriolar phenotype is propagated in the downstream capillaries, priming them for further enlargement, stimulation of smooth muscle cells proliferation, etc.

Two important observations should be made: a) The incorporation of CPEC into capillaries at the arteriolar side may contribute to the extension of arterioles (particularly if CPEC start to proliferate). This is related to the recent observation that in the stretch-induced angiogenesis of striated muscle, growth of arterioles precedes that of capillaries[48]. b) This angiogenic mechanism is different from sprouting, where the *original* EC of a microvessel, usually believed to be a venule[49], proliferate, migrate, etc.

We did not address the process of capillary formation in first place, or the extension of venules, two instances which remain open for explanations based on the sprouting model. Sprouting of capillaries on one side, and the engraftment of CPEC in extracellular matrix or in arteriolar extensions on another side, may be conceived as compatible or even complementary processes, within the framework of the tunneling model.

The suggested mechanism of CPEC engraftment may also apply for those situations where there are no true capillaries involved, but only tunnels. Therefore, from the point of view of the tissular insemination of CPEC the process looks similar, and may be summated in the same tunneling mechanism (Fig. 5). This is also shown in the cartoon presented in Fig. 6, where the capillaries and/or the tunnels would act as "retention filters" for CPEC recruitment. The model suggests an explanation for the transformation of the progenitors in more mature circulating EC[50]. CPEC would spend some time in capillaries,

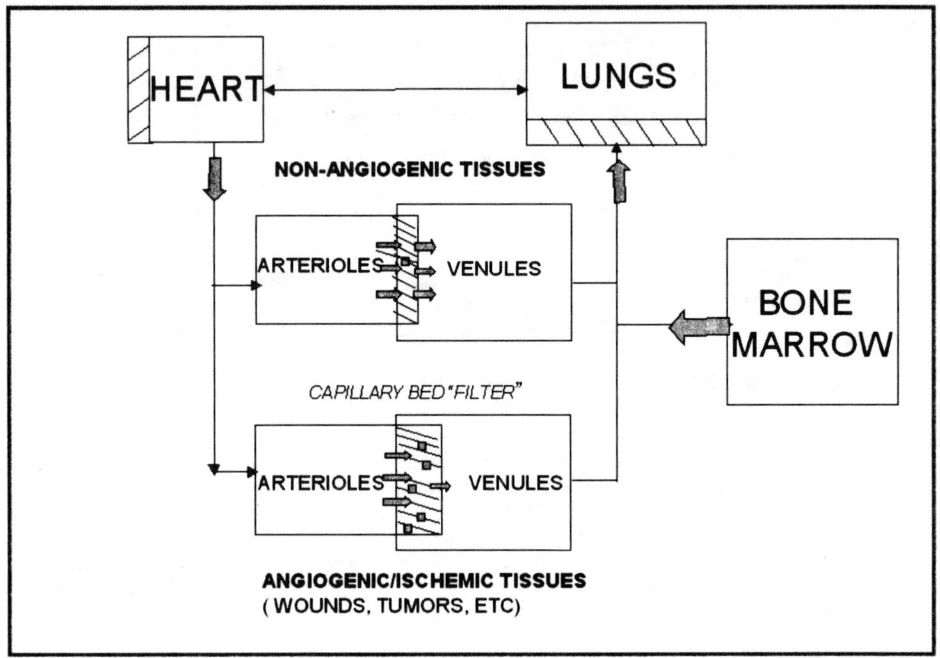

Figure 6. A model of CPEC recruitment at angiogenic foci. In non-angiogenic vascular beds, CPEC originated from the bone marrow would undergo repeated passing without retention. In angiogenic tissues, as part of the inflammatory infiltrate, CPEC would be trapped in adherent capillaries, or in tunnels created by monocytes/macrophages. Alternatively, CPEC may be simply slowed down during their passage, but the extended exposure to local angiogenic milieu would induce their differentiation in more mature circulating EC, until they finally stop and engraft.

where they might have time and local conditions to mature, and if they do not adhere to the lumen, they keep cycling with the blood throughout the circulation, where they are detected as more "mature" EC (see also Mancuso et al., Chapter 9 of this volume). These cells may also be shed, or lost through apoptosis, from a bona fide endothelium, through an yet to be defined mechanism.

A final comment is to be made, regarding the generality of the tunneling model in its restraint (monocyte/macrophage based) sense. Does it apply only to the inflammatory angiogenesis? Maybe not, considering that there are ubiquitous tissular macrophages, even in very small numbers, which might perform the tunneling function described here. As discussed before, these non-endothelial cells are known to be involved in the sprouting-based angiogenesis[12].

8. CONCLUSIONS

In this paper we have defined and recapitulated several steps in the development of the concept of tunneling. We also presented its applications related to the tissular insemination of CPEC. In this model, the penetration of extracellular matrix by CPEC and by advancing capillary tips, or both, may benefit from the proteolytic activity of more potent co-migrating cells, in particular monocytes/macrophages. The same concept could explain re-canalization of clots, where blood flow in parallel with the original lumen may be re-established by the inflammatory cells. These cells have the ability to produce tunnels in the extracellular matrices and cover and/or fill them, and to accommodate other cells as well. Furthermore, if among these co-localized cells are CPEC, they may colonize the tunnels and contribute later to their transformation into microvessels[26].

Finally, we discussed an analogy between the localization of CPEC in tunnels and in capillaries, as a common pattern of behavior of these cells. This is suggestive for the mechanism of propagation of arteriolar phenotype into the downstream capillary beds, in active angiogenic fields.

The tunneling hypothesis and its applications need more experimental evidence, a task actively pursued in our laboratory. Nevertheless, it already offers an attractive conceptual framework for the explanation of a number of observations regarding the intercellular cooperation on bio-mechanical grounds, particularly in the field of adult angiogenesis.

9. ACKNOWLEDGEMENTS

This presentation incorporates work done by Mirela Anghelina, MD, Padma Krishnan, MS, Leni Moldovan, PhD, Somil Gupta, MBBS and Sumant Kulkarni, MS. The author is also grateful to Dr. P. Goldschmidt-Clermont for advice in the early stages of this project, and Drs. P. E. Kolattukudy, R. Altschuld and C. Leier for providing the mouse, rat and human specimens, respectively. This work was supported by a Beginning Grant in Aid from the American Heart Association, Ohio Affiliate, and by the NIH grant R01 HL65983.

10. REFERENCES

1. T.Asahara, T.Murohara, A.Sullivan, M.Silver, Z.R.van der, T.Li, B.Witzenbichler, G.Schatteman, and J.M.Isner, Isolation of putative progenitor endothelial cells for angiogenesis, *Science* **275**(5302), 964-967 (1997).
2. T.Takahashi, C.Kalka, H.Masuda, D.Chen, M.Silver, M.Kearney, M.Magner, J.M.Isner, and T.Asahara, Ischemia- and cytokine-induced mobilization of bone marrow-derived endothelial progenitor cells for neovascularization, *Nat. Med.* **5**(4), 434-438 (1999).
3. G.C.Schatteman, H.D.Hanlon, C.Jiao, S.G.Dodds, and B.A.Christy, Blood-derived angioblasts accelerate blood-flow restoration in diabetic mice, *J. Clin. Invest* **106**(4), 571-578 (2000).
4. S.Rafii, Circulating endothelial precursors: mystery, reality, and promise, *J. Clin. Invest* **105**(1), 17-19 (2000).
5. E.Gunsilius, H.C.Duba, A.L.Petzer, C.M.Kahler, K.Grunewald, G.Stockhammer, C.Gabl, S.Dirnhofer, J.Clausen, and G.Gastl, Evidence from a leukaemia model for maintenance of vascular endothelium by bone-marrow-derived endothelial cells, *Lancet* **355**(9216), 1688-1691 (2000).
6. T.Graf, Differentiation plasticity of hematopoietic cells, *Blood* **99**(9), 3089-3101 (2002).
7. B.Alberts, D.Bray, J.Lewis, M.Raff, K.Roberts, and J.D.Watson, *Molecular Biology of the Cell. 3rd Ed*, (Garland Science Publishing, New York).

8.   S.M.Schwartz, C.M.Gajdusek, M.A.Reidy, S.C.Selden, III, and C.C.Haudenschild, Maintenance of integrity in aortic endothelium, *Fed. Proc.* **39**(9), 2618-2625 (1980).

9.   J.Folkman and C.Haudenschild, Angiogenesis by capillary endothelial cells in culture, *Trans. Ophthalmol. Soc. U. K.* **100**(3), 346-353 (1980).

10. M.M.Sholley, G.P.Ferguson, H.R.Seibel, J.L.Montour, and J.D.Wilson, Mechanisms of neovascularization. Vascular sprouting can occur without proliferation of endothelial cells, *Lab Invest* **51**(6), 624-634 (1984).

11. P.Libby and U.Schonbeck, Drilling for oxygen: angiogenesis involves proteolysis of the extracellular matrix, *Circ. Res.* **89**(3), 195-197 (2001).

12. L.Diaz-Flores, R.Gutierrez, and H.Varela, Behavior of postcapillary venule pericytes during postnatal angiogenesis, *J. Morphol.* **213**(1), 33-45 (1992).

13. V.Nehls, K.Denzer, and D.Drenckhahn, Pericyte involvement in capillary sprouting during angiogenesis in situ, *Cell Tissue Res.* **270**(3), 469-474 (1992).

14. H.Tsuzuki and S.Sasa, Ultrastructural observation of capillary sprouts in the dental organs of rat molars, *Kaibogaku Zasshi* **69**(5), 684-696 (1994).

15. A.Sasaki, Y.Nakazato, A.Ogawa, and S.Sugihara, The immunophenotype of perivascular cells in the human brain, *Pathol. Int.* **46**(1), 15-23 (1996).

16. L.Diaz-Flores, R.Gutierrez, A.Lopez-Alonso, R.Gonzalez, and H.Varela, Pericytes as a supplementary source of osteoblasts in periosteal osteogenesis, *Clin. Orthop.*275), 280-286 (1992).

17. J.R.Crosby, W.E.Kaminski, G.Schatteman, P.J.Martin, E.W.Raines, R.A.Seifert, and D.F.Bowen-Pope, Endothelial cells of hematopoietic origin make a significant contribution to adult blood vessel formation, *Circ. Res* **87**(9), 728-730 (2000).

18. M.Reyes, A.Dudek, B.Jahagirdar, L.Koodie, P.H.Marker, and C.M.Verfaillie, Origin of endothelial progenitors in human postnatal bone marrow, *J. Clin. Invest* **109**(3), 337-346 (2002).

19. M.Harraz, C.Jiao, H.D.Hanlon, R.S.Hartley, and G.C.Schatteman, Cd34(-) blood-derived human endothelial cell progenitors, *Stem Cells* **19**(4), 304-312 (2001).

20. J.M.Isner, C.Kalka, A.Kawamoto, and T.Asahara, Bone marrow as a source of endothelial cells for natural and iatrogenic vascular repair, *Ann. N. Y. Acad. Sci.* **953**(75-84 (2001).

21. Dahlqvist k, E.Y.Umemoto, J.J.Brokaw, M.Dupuis, and D.M.McDonald, Tissue macrophages associated with angiogenesis in chronic airway inflammation in rats, *Am. J. Respir. Cell Mol. Biol.* **20**(2), 237-247 (1999).

22. M.Madlener, W.C.Parks, and S.Werner, Matrix metalloproteinases (MMPs) and their physiological inhibitors (TIMPs) are differentially expressed during excisional skin wound repair, *Exp. Cell Res.* **242**(1), 201-210 (1998).

23. G.T.Meyer, L.J.Matthias, L.Noack, M.A.Vadas, and J.R.Gamble, Lumen formation during angiogenesis in vitro involves phagocytic activity, formation and secretion of vacuoles, cell death, and capillary tube remodelling by different populations of endothelial cells, *Anat. Rec.* **249**(3), 327-340 (1997).

24. J.M.Isner and T.Asahara, Angiogenesis and vasculogenesis as therapeutic strategies for postnatal neovascularization, *J. Clin. Invest* **103**(9), 1231-1236 (1999).

25. N.I.Moldovan, P.J.Goldschmidt-Clermont, J.Parker-Thornburg, S.D.Shapiro, and P.E.Kolattukudy, Contribution of monocytes/macrophages to compensatory neovascularization: the drilling of metalloelastase-positive tunnels in ischemic myocardium, *Circ. Res.* **87**(5), 378-384 (2000).

26. Moldovan, NI. Role of monocytes and macrophages in adult angiogenesis: a light at the tunnel'e end. J Hematother Stem Cell Res . 2002.

27. L.F.Brown, A.M.Dvorak, and H.F.Dvorak, Leaky vessels, fibrin deposition, and fibrosis: a sequence of events common to solid tumors and to many other types of disease, *Am. Rev. Respir. Dis.* **140**(4), 1104-1107 (1989).

28. N.I.Moldovan, Z.Qian, Y.Chen, C.Dong, A.Ying, R.H.Hruban, N.A.Flavahan, W.M.Baldwin III, F.Sanfilippo, and P.J.Goldschmidt-Clermont, Fas-mediated apoptosis in accelerated graft arteriosclerosis, *Angiogenesis* **2**(3), 245-254 (2002).

29. P.E.Kolattukudy, T.Quach, S.Bergese, S.Breckenridge, J.Hensley, R.Altschuld, G.Gordillo, S.Klenotic, C.Orosz, and J.Parker-Thornburg, Myocarditis induced by targeted expression of the MCP-1 gene in murine cardiac muscle, *Am. J. Pathol.* **152**(1), 101-111 (1998).

30. C.M.Hohl, B.Hu, R.H.Fertel, J.C.Russell, S.A.McCune, and R.A.Altschuld, Effects of obesity and hypertension on ventricular myocytes: comparison of cells from adult SHHF/Mcc-cp and JCR:LA-cp rats, *Cardiovasc. Res.* **27**(2), 238-242 (1993).

31. M.Terashima, K.Awano, Y.Honda, N.Yoshino, T.Mori, H.Fujita, Y.Ohashi, O.Seguchi, K.Kobayashi, M.Yamagishi, P.J.Fitzgerald, P.G.Yock, and K.Maeda, Images in cardiovascular medicine. "Arter-

ies within the artery" after Kawasaki disease: a lotus root appearance by intravascular ultrasound, *Circulation* **106**(7), 887 (2002).

32. M.Adachi, S.Suematsu, T.Suda, D.Watanabe, H.Fukuyama, J.Ogasawara, T.Tanaka, N.Yoshida, and S.Nagata, Enhanced and accelerated lymphoproliferation in Fas-null mice, *Proc. Natl. Acad. Sci. U. S. A* **93**(5), 2131-2136 (1996).

33. V.Bhattacharya, P.A.McSweeney, Q.Shi, B.Bruno, A.Ishida, R.Nash, R.F.Storb, L.R.Sauvage, W.P.Hammond, and M.H.Wu, Enhanced endothelialization and microvessel formation in polyester grafts seeded with CD34(+) bone marrow cells, *Blood* **95**(2), 581-585 (2000).

34. Q.Shi, M.H.Wu, Y.Fujita, A.Ishida, E.S.Wijelath, W.P.Hammond, A.R.Wechezak, C.Yu, R.F.Storb, and L.R.Sauvage, Genetic tracing of arterial graft flow surface endothelialization in allogeneic marrow transplanted dogs, *Cardiovasc. Surg.* **7**(1), 98-105 (1999).

35. B.Peault, I.L.Weissman, A.M.Buckle, A.Tsukamoto, and C.Baum, Thy-1-expressing CD34+ human cells express multiple hematopoietic potentialities in vitro and in SCID-hu mice, *Nouv. Rev. Fr. Hematol.* **35**(1), 91-93 (1993).

36. W.S.Lee, M.K.Jain, B.M.Arkonac, D.Zhang, S.Y.Shaw, S.Kashiki, K.Maemura, S.L.Lee, N.K.Hollenberg, M.E.Lee, and E.Haber, Thy-1, a novel marker for angiogenesis upregulated by inflammatory cytokines, *Circ. Res.* **82**(8), 845-851 (1998).

37. H.F.Dvorak, V.S.Harvey, P.Estrella, L.F.Brown, J.McDonagh, and A.M.Dvorak, Fibrin containing gels induce angiogenesis. Implications for tumor stroma generation and wound healing, *Lab Invest* **57**(6), 673-686 (1987).

38. D.M.McDonald, L.Munn, and R.K.Jain, Vasculogenic mimicry: how convincing, how novel, and how significant?, *Am. J. Pathol.* **156**(2), 383-388 (2000).

39. T.M.Schlaeger, S.Bartunkova, J.A.Lawitts, G.Teichmann, W.Risau, U.Deutsch, and T.N.Sato, Uniform vascular-endothelial-cell-specific gene expression in both embryonic and adult transgenic mice, *Proc. Natl. Acad. Sci. U. S. A* **94**(7), 3058-3063 (1997).

40. T.Asahara, T.Takahashi, H.Masuda, C.Kalka, D.Chen, H.Iwaguro, Y.Inai, M.Silver, and J.M.Isner, VEGF contributes to postnatal neovascularization by mobilizing bone marrow-derived endothelial progenitor cells, *EMBO J.* **18**(14), 3964-3972 (1999).

41. A.Passaniti, R.M.Taylor, R.Pili, Y.Guo, P.V.Long, J.A.Haney, R.R.Pauly, D.S.Grant, and G.R.Martin, A simple, quantitative method for assessing angiogenesis and antiangiogenic agents using reconstituted basement membrane, heparin, and fibroblast growth factor, *Lab Invest* **67**(4), 519-528 (1992).

42. S.Gordon, Macrophage-restricted molecules: role in differentiation and activation, *Immunol. Lett.* **65**(1-2), 5-8 (1999).

43. V.Nehls, R.Herrmann, and M.Huhnken, Guided migration as a novel mechanism of capillary network remodeling is regulated by basic fibroblast growth factor, *Histochem. Cell Biol.* **109**(4), 319-329 (1998).

44. D.B.Archer and T.A.Gardiner, Electron microscopic features of experimental choroidal neovascularization, *Am. J. Ophthalmol.* **91**(4), 433-457 (1981).

45. N.W.Gale, P.Baluk, L.Pan, M.Kwan, J.Holash, T.M.DeChiara, D.M.McDonald, and G.D.Yancopoulos, Ephrin-B2 selectively marks arterial vessels and neovascularization sites in the adult, with expression in both endothelial and smooth- muscle cells, *Dev. Biol.* **230**(2), 151-160 (2001).

46. M.A.Rupnick, D.Panigrahy, C.Y.Zhang, S.M.Dallabrida, B.B.Lowell, R.Langer, and M.J.Folkman, Adipose tissue mass can be regulated through the vasculature, *Proc. Natl. Acad. Sci. U. S. A* **99**(16), 10730-10735 (2002).

47. M.Nesbit, H.Schaider, T.H.Miller, and M.Herlyn, Low-level monocyte chemoattractant protein-1 stimulation of monocytes leads to tumor formation in nontumorigenic melanoma cells, *J. Immunol.* **166**(11), 6483-6490 (2001).

48. F.Hansen-Smith, S.Egginton, A.L.Zhou, and O.Hudlicka, Growth of arterioles precedes that of capillaries in stretch-induced angiogenesis in skeletal muscle, *Microvasc. Res.* **62**(1), 1-14 (2001).

49. K.Yuan, Y.T.Jin, and M.T.Lin, Expression of Tie-2, angiopoietin-1, angiopoietin-2, ephrinB2 and EphB4 in pyogenic granuloma of human gingiva implicates their roles in inflammatory angiogenesis, *J. Periodontal Res.* **35**(3), 165-171 (2000).

50. S.Monestiroli, P.Mancuso, A.Burlini, G.Pruneri, C.Dell'Agnola, A.Gobbi, G.Martinelli, and F.Bertolini, Kinetics and viability of circulating endothelial cells as surrogate angiogenesis marker in an animal model of human lymphoma, *Cancer Res.* **61** (11), 4341-4344 (2001).

INDEX

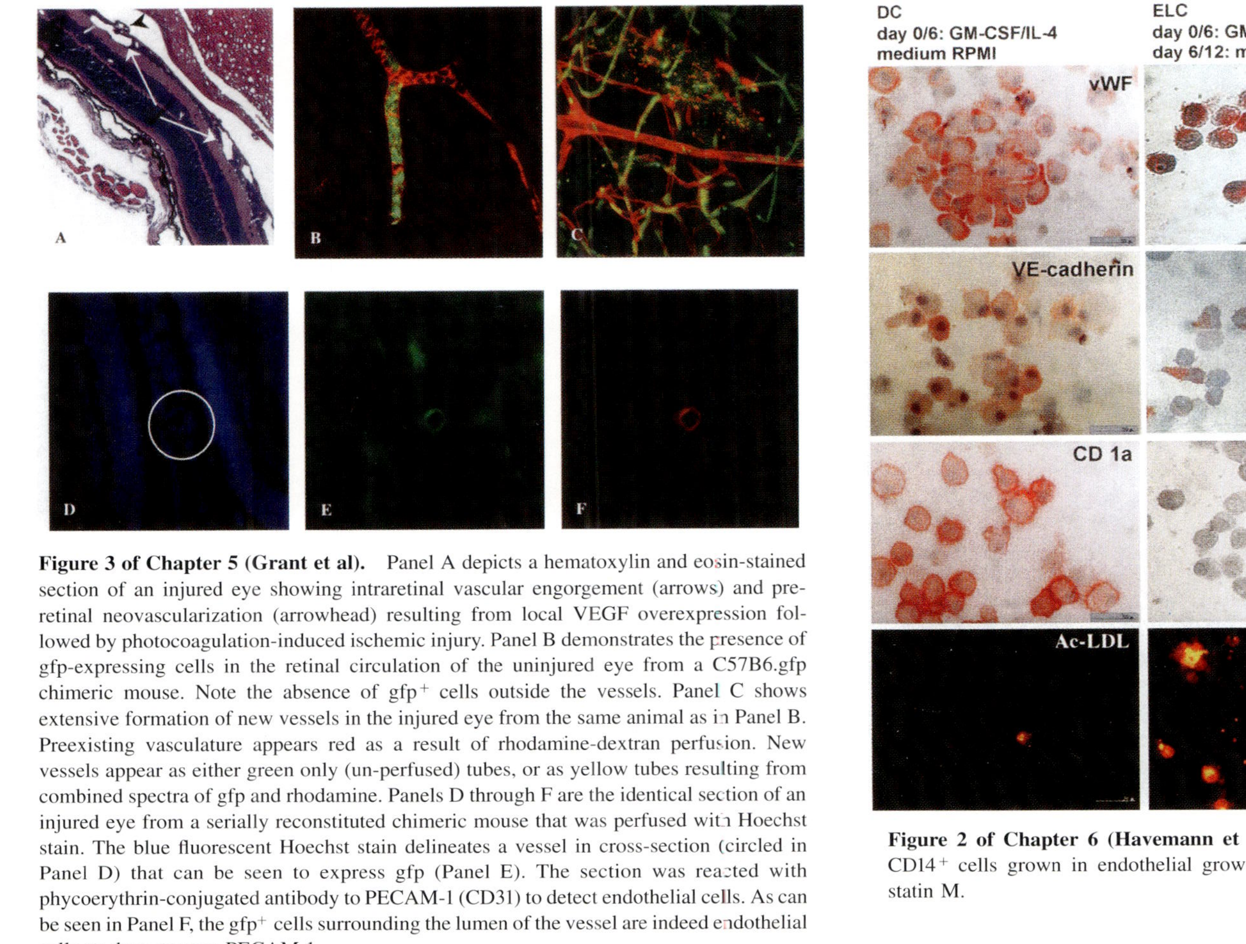

Figure 3 of Chapter 5 (Grant et al).   Panel A depicts a hematoxylin and eosin-stained section of an injured eye showing intraretinal vascular engorgement (arrows) and pre-retinal neovascularization (arrowhead) resulting from local VEGF overexpression followed by photocoagulation-induced ischemic injury. Panel B demonstrates the presence of gfp-expressing cells in the retinal circulation of the uninjured eye from a C57B6.gfp chimeric mouse. Note the absence of gfp+ cells outside the vessels. Panel C shows extensive formation of new vessels in the injured eye from the same animal as in Panel B. Preexisting vasculature appears red as a result of rhodamine-dextran perfusion. New vessels appear as either green only (un-perfused) tubes, or as yellow tubes resulting from combined spectra of gfp and rhodamine. Panels D through F are the identical section of an injured eye from a serially reconstituted chimeric mouse that was perfused with Hoechst stain. The blue fluorescent Hoechst stain delineates a vessel in cross-section (circled in Panel D) that can be seen to express gfp (Panel E). The section was reacted with phycoerythrin-conjugated antibody to PECAM-1 (CD31) to detect endothelial cells. As can be seen in Panel F, the gfp+ cells surrounding the lumen of the vessel are indeed endothelial cells as they express PECAM-1.

Figure 2 of Chapter 6 (Havemann et al.).   Immunohistochemical characterisation of CD14+ cells grown in endothelial growth medium supplemented with IL-4 and onco-statin M.

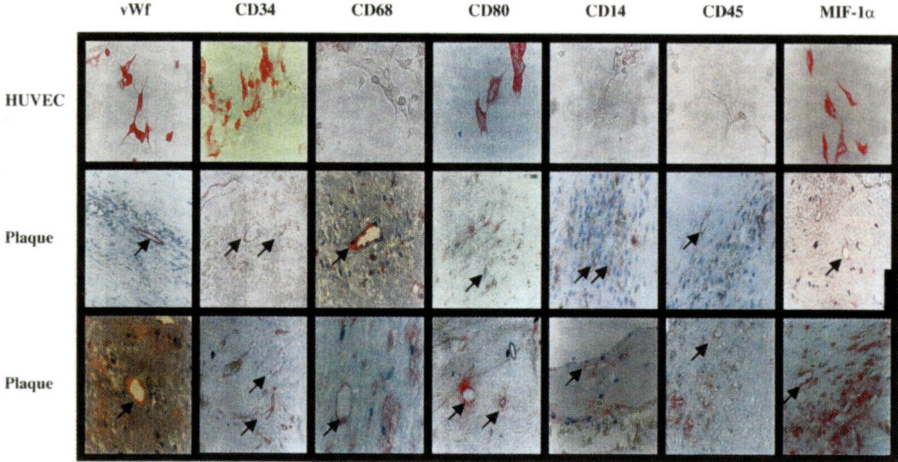

Figure 3 of Chapter 7 (Schmeisser et al.).   In vivo equivalent for ECs with phenotypical overlap to monocytes/ macrophages. Histological examination of microvascular endothelial cells within neovascularized advanced human atherosclerotic plaques. (Original magnification × 200). HUVECs, stimulated by TNF-α (10ng/ml) were used as controls. (Original magnification × 100) (from Schmeisser, paper in preparation).

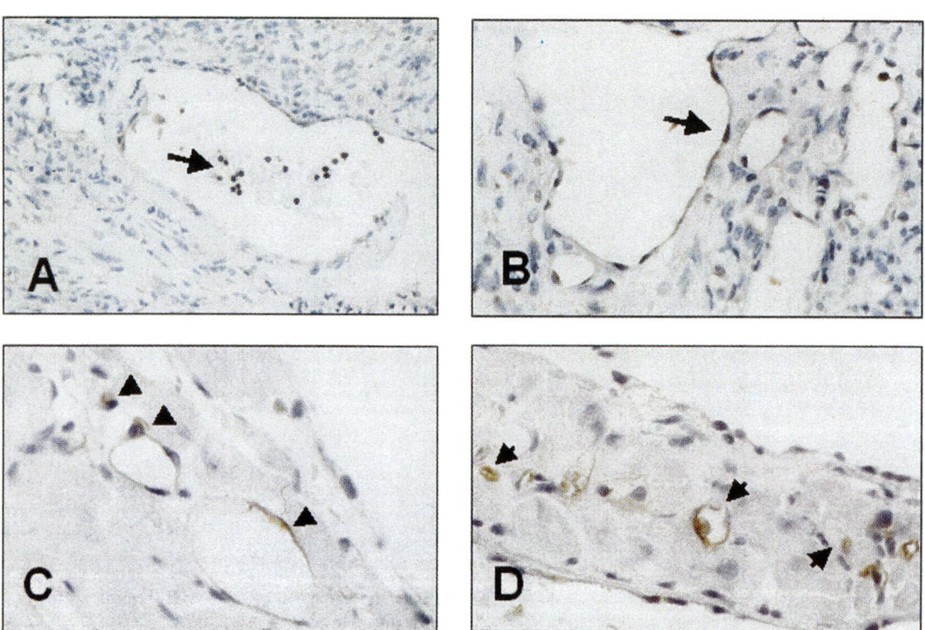

Figure 3 of Chapter 10 (Moldovan).   Contribution of CPEC to neo-vascularization in adult animals. A, B. Recipient blood-derived mononuclear cells engrafting in the intimal layer of a transplanted mouse heart. The images represent immunostaining for the Fas marker, present only in the cells of the recipient animal. A. Fas-positive leukocytes (arrow) are aggregated in a clot in the lumen of a microvessel from the Fas-deficient (lpr) transplanted heart. Note that in this section the endothelium of the transplanted vessel is negative for Fas. B. Another section in the same lpr transplant, shows Fas-positive cells in an endothelial position (arrow) and Fas-positive infiltrating mononuclear cells. C, D. Expression of the hematopoietic marker Thy-1 (arrowheads) in neo-angiogenic fields in failing MCP-1 hearts (C) and in SHHF rats (D). In C, the distributions of positive cells relative to the lumen of a microvessel (outside, tangential, luminal) suggest a stepwise incorporation from the outside. A–D, hematoxylin counterstaining. Original magnifications, ×120.